THE CHOLESTEROL CONTROVERSY

PUBLISHER'S NOTE

On January 3, 1973, after the text of this book was set in type, the Federal Trade Commission (FTC) publicly announced its complaint and order to the manufacturer of, and advertising agency for Fleischmann's margarine to cease and desist in making health claims for that product. In an agreement between the FTC and Standard Brands, Inc., Fleischmann's margarine, **"or any other margarine or any other food fat or food oil,"** is prohibited from making any claim that such a product (which stresses its polyunsaturated fat content) will prevent or mitigate heart and artery disease. The FTC complaint stated that such advertising is "unfair and deceptive" and is "to the prejudice and injury of the public." In addition, the FTC stated that because there is no competent and reliable evidence to show that premature heart and artery disease during adult life is caused by childhood diet, Fleischmann's margarine may no longer advertise any connection between childhood diet and adult heart disease. Violation of this order may result in a civil penalty up to $5,000 per violation. This action by the FTC, the first of its kind after more than two years of investigation, definitively supports and further documents the subject matter of this book.

Cholesterol

CHOLESTEROL, A 27-CARBON COMPOUND, IS SYNTHESIZED in man by a process of more than thirty steps, after acetate has been activated by an enzyme into acetyl coenzyme-A. The liver is the most important site of cholesterol biosynthesis and the intestinal tract is another important site. The cholesterol in serum probably does not contribute much toward the formation of cholesterol-rich cell membranes, for most of the body's cells produce pure cholesterol. Its presence in structural elements, red cells, and plasma accounts for the fact that cholesterol is abundant in the body. It is only exceeded in serum by phospholipids.

THE CHOLESTEROL CONTROVERSY

Edward R. Pinckney, M.D.
Cathey Pinckney

Sherbourne Press   Los Angeles

Published by Sherbourne Press, Inc., 1640 So. La Cienega Blvd.
Los Angeles, Ca 90035
Second Printing
Library of Congress Catalog Card Number 72-96515
ISBN 0-8202-0155-3
Composition   Datagraphics, Phoenix, Arizona
Printed and bound by Levison-McNally, Reno, Nev.

ACKNOWLEDGEMENTS

We wish to acknowledge the following people, without whose stimulus this book would never have been written.

Forrest H. Adams, M.D., Past President of the American College of Cardiology.

Henry W. Blackburn, Jr., M.D., Lecturer, Department of Medicine, University of Minnesota.

Douglas C. Fisk, Manager, Dairy Council of California.

Ernest B. Howard, M.D., Executive Vice President of the American Medical Association.

Donald N. Kilburn, Assistant to the Director, Division of Regulatory Operations, Office of Compliance, Bureau of Drugs, Food and Drug Administration.

Daniel Melnick, Ph.D., Vice President, Corn Products International, Inc.

R. E. Newberry, Assistant to the Director, Division of Regulatory Guidance, Office of Compliance, Bureau of Foods, Food and Drug Administration.

Jeremiah Stamler, M.D., of the Chicago Health Research Foundation and Member of the Council on Epidemiology of the American Heart Association.

Frederick J. Stare, M.D., Department of Nutrition, Harvard University.

Malcolm R. Stephens, Past President, Institution of Shortening and Edible Oils, Inc.

Sidney Weissenberg, Division of Scientific Opinions, Federal Trade Commission.

The "Letters to Harvey," in the introduction to Chapter 10, are reproduced with the permission of the author, Frederick L. Jones, Jr., M.D., and the publishers of *Medical Opinion*, where they first appeared.

CONTENTS

All human history attests
That happiness for man—the hungry sinner—
Since Eve ate apples, much depends on dinner.
Lord Byron

PART **I**

AT THE HEART
OF THE DILEMMA

YOU ARE LONGING for a fluffy omelette, or perhaps a hamburger and a milkshake, but you have a nagging fear that these foods might be bad for your heart. So, you forego your heart's desire, as well as foods that contain cholesterol, and silently but unnecessarily suffer. Thanks almost solely to "Madison Avenue" promotion by certain commercial food producers and the American Heart Association, a great many people imagine that if they lower their blood cholesterol—assuming it is elevated—they will prevent heart disease, heart attacks, and even treat any heart trouble they may now have. At the same time, most people do not know the whole truth about cholesterol testing, what cholesterol really is, or the importance of cholesterol to body function. Few people realize that there has never been a proven, scientific relationship between lowering blood cholesterol levels and preventing heart disease. Even if you could lower the amount of cholesterol that can be measured in your blood, there is no proof that you will, in any way, reduce your chances for a heart attack.

CHAPTER *1*

LET THE CONSUMER
BE WARY

YOUR FEAR OF dying—if you happen to be one of the great many people who suffer from this morbid preoccupation—may well have made you a victim of the cholesterol controversy. For, if you have come to believe that you can ward off death from heart disease by altering the amount of cholesterol in your blood, whether by diet or by drugs, you are following a regime that still has no basis in fact. Rather, you as a consumer, have been taken in by certain commercial interests and health groups who are more interested in your money than your life.

No matter what you have seen or heard to the contrary, there is absolutely *no* scientific evidence to prove that even if you could consistently lower the amount of cholesterol in your blood, as measured by a laboratory test, you would decrease your chances of having a heart attack. Nor has anyone proved that you could prevent some form of heart or artery disease from starting, or from progressing, if it already exists. But, if you enjoy fine food, you may be making yourself miserable three times a day without purpose.

There are quite a number of scientific experiments to show that an increase in polyunsaturates in your diet, for the purpose of lowering blood cholesterol, may cause you to appear much older than you are (premature aging), an increased amount of cancers, and a host of other damaging diseases. In spite of the fact that there is medical evidence of potential dangers from eating an excess of polyunsaturates, these particular fats and oils are being extensively, albeit illegally, advertised and promoted as "medicines" for the heart with no warning notice of those potentially dangerous side-effects. Thus, the consumer's understandable fear of heart disease and an impending early death is being exploited by certain health groups as well as by an industry whose profits have more than doubled as a direct result of its implied promise that heart disease and death can be forestalled through the use of its products.

The very word "polyunsaturated" has become synonymous with protection against heart disease, just as the words "cholesterol" or "saturated fat" have been made to intimate doom. Although the federal government, through the Food and Drug Administration (FDA) has officially stated since 1959 (and even reaffirmed its prohibitive doctrine in 1964 and 1971) that it is a violation of the law to advertise polyunsaturates as a "drug" to prevent or treat heart disease, to this date it has never enforced that law. Another government agency, the Federal Trade Commission (FTC), has admitted that for years it has "investigated" advertising that makes unwarranted heart disease protection claims for highly polyunsaturated foods, and has publicly promised action on such unproved health claims, but it, too, has done nothing to date.

Consumer Reports magazine, as far back as its May, 1963, issue deplored "The promotion of margarine as a drug." This publication also openly attacked the Food and Drug Administration for not matching its words with its deeds, when the government agency refused to enforce its own laws against polyunsaturate advertising founded on "false, fear-based claims." Now, of course, a margarine or oil advertiser does not have to go any further than to mention its polyunsaturate content for the public to draw the conclusion that the product is still primarily for health purposes. Consumer's Union concluded that "the amounts of unsaturated fat available to the diet through margarine cannot be considered significant." They further concluded that the main result of polyunsaturate promotion is profit to the manufacturer.

The conspiracy to force certain fats and oils on the public

for health purposes has been condemned by Dr. George V. Mann, professor of medicine at Vanderbilt University, who calls the emphasis on cholesterol lowering a "wasteful diversion" and then goes so far as to say: "The vegetable oil industry, with some help from science adventurists, has taken the citizenry down the garden path on this unsaturated fat issue."

Scientists of the Agricultural Research Service have reported to the U.S. Senate's Agricultural Appropriations Subcommittee that corn oil, which is pointedly advertised to reduce cholesterol, actually causes more cholesterol to be produced by the body than does butterfat or beef fat. The nutritionists who conducted the study emphasized the absolute need for further investigation before *any* dietary changes are recommended as a means of reducing cholesterol. In 1972, these findings were reaffirmed by Dr. W. O. Caster and his associates at the University of Georgia. They found that the *more* stearates (the fatty acid of meat fats) that were eaten, the *lower* the blood cholesterol went. As an incidental finding, it was noted that blood pressure also was reduced when meat fat was part of the diet.

During the past two decades the "average" American has increased his consumption of polyunsaturates to three times the quantity that was eaten back in the 1940's. At the same time he has reduced his intake of dairy foods, eggs, beef, and pork to less than half. And, with all this, the heart disease rate has climbed almost parallel to the rise in polyunsaturates in the diet. Certainly if polyunsaturates really did work as claimed, with the millions of people purposely eating so much of these particular fats, we should have had *some* reduction in heart attacks. But instead all forms of heart disease have actually skyrocketed!

Since medical science has not, as yet, even come close to proving that cholesterol in the blood is the cause of heart disease, it becomes ridiculous to postulate that altering the amount of cholesterol in one's blood, especially through diet, will make any difference in the health of one's heart. Yet government agencies have allowed health associations and food industries to play havoc with the anxieties of millions and millions of people by permitting this unproved doctrine to be promoted.

The commercial stress on the use of polyunsaturates to lower blood cholesterol as a means of protecting the heart is probably the greatest single factor holding back research into truly effective means of preventing and curing heart disease. Moreover, the public is being motivated by fear tactics into a diet regime that may be more harmful than helpful; it is pleasure lost with nothing gained.

CHAPTER 2

PITFALLS OF MEASURING
YOUR BLOOD CHOLESTEROL

THE AVERAGE MAN and woman has come to believe that should a medical laboratory test show that the cholesterol in his or her blood is numerically greater than it is supposed to be, life's ultimate catastrophe is imminent. Although there are many factors involved in bringing on heart disease, the fear-provoking factor that is most blatantly being promoted to the American consumer is the dire consequence that may result from an elevated blood (or serum, or plasma) cholesterol. That a simple laboratory test to show the amount of cholesterol in the blood should be fraught with such fear is the result of some extremely successful commercial maneuvering and not a little dissembling. Every time the consumer opens a magazine or newspaper, turns on the radio or television, some commercial or advertisement tells him to buy this or that product because it is low in cholesterol, or that it will lower his cholesterol and therefore be good for his heart. What those who promote these hypotheses are reluctant to talk about are the many divergent scientific opinions and findings.

Dr. William B. Kannel, director of the now famous "Framingham Study" (a study that hoped to reveal the primary risks of heart attack), once said that a blood test for cholesterol was probably the most useful measure to show existing or even impending heart disease. Thousands of men and women in the city of Framingham, Massachusetts were then studied to try and relate heart disease to any and all theorized causes. But, after fourteen years, all that was really discovered was that half of the people in the study who did die of a heart attack had offered *no* prior laboratory evidence (elevated blood cholesterol) that would have raised any alarm that they had pre-existing heart disease. Furthermore, there was absolutely *no* relationship found between what a person ate and the level of his blood cholesterol.

In another similar study of 500 patients in Seattle, Washington, only one out of every 25 people (only 4 percent) who had a heart attack, had an elevated cholesterol.

Dr. Robert I. Levy, chief of the National Heart and Lung Institute's Lipid Metabolism Branch (the federal government's primary facility for cholesterol studies) stated in 1971: "We don't know that lowering cholesterol [as measured by a laboratory test] will decrease the rate and risk of heart disease."

Dr. Edward H. Ahrens, professor at the Rockefeller University in New York City has said: "Plasma cholesterol levels are a very unreliable indicator of what's happening in the body."

Such authoritative medical opinions must not be forgotten or ignored when those who, for their own profit, urge you to think otherwise.

Probably the most unique circumstance of all, when it comes to measuring blood cholesterol, is that this particular test is subject to more errors and variations than almost any other laboratory procedure. As a simple example, if you are only slightly "upset" at having a laboratory test performed—either because the sticking of a needle in your arm to take your blood bothers you, or because you already fear that the test to measure how much cholesterol you have floating about in your bloodstream might imply you have heart disease—then, the result of that cholesterol test taken at that particular time could be wrong by as much as 100 percent. Whereas you might well have a cholesterol level of 200 mg. percent* which is well within today's so-called normal limits), fear, anxiety or apprehension can raise

---

* Blood cholesterol levels are reported as so many milligrams for each 100 ml. (3 1/3 ounces) of blood. For example, a blood cholesterol of 200 means 200 mg. for each 100 ml. of blood, sometimes reported as mg. percent (mg. %). Most blood tests are transposed to mg. percent so as to have a common standard.

your cholesterol level so that the laboratory test will come out to be 400—enough to make you (and possibly your doctor) start the vicious cycle of "treating" potential heart disease with all the restrictive measures conjured up by the possibility of heart disease. But, it has also been shown that the same test performed without the direct knowledge of the patient that it allegedly stands for an ominous warning of heart disease—especially when the normal anticipation that comes from needles has been alleviated—can yield a number that is well below what is, at this time, considered to be "dangerous."

That the "mood" you are in at the moment your blood is taken to measure your cholesterol is important, can be demonstrated by the fact that cholesterol tests performed only hours apart on the same patient show differences of more than 100. In one patient, cholesterol tests were performed on a so-called "routine" basis and a difference of more than 200 was found on two consecutive days. If, while you are reading this, you become apprehensive, you are, no doubt, momentarily raising your cholesterol level. If, on the other hand, you are finding some comfort and support in the fact that cholesterol tests are not that accurate, let alone that prognostic, you could actually be lowering your cholesterol level.

How fast can your emotions alter your cholesterol level? Think back on the time, when lying in bed late one evening, you suddenly awoke and *thought* you heard a strange noise in some other part of the house. How long did it take for you to realize your heart was pounding faster and that you were covered with a cold sweat? No more than a few seconds. Your mind "interpreted" the sounds (if you really recognized what they were immediately, you would not have panicked) and translated your "imagined" fear to your endocrine glands. Even before you could reason out what the sounds were, the hormones in your body had started to act. The same thing applies to your blood cholesterol level. Fear, apprehension, even a vivid imagination, can release hormones in your body that will instantaneously elevate your cholesterol level along with many other chemicals in the bloodstream. And, while you may get over your momentary anxiety within a short time, it can take hours for your body level of cholesterol to return to its previous lower value.

So keep these facts in mind as you delve into the mysteries

of how blood cholesterol is measured and what it really means insofar as disease is concerned.

The history of the changes in the interpretation of cholesterol values is in itself unique. In 1950 a blood cholesterol level greater than 150 was considered pathological. By 1970 new discoveries regarding normal changes with age were such that a value of 300 was, in most instances, considered within the range of normal.

Before blood cholesterol measurements became so intimately involved with potential heart disease—albeit still only hypothetically—the amount of cholesterol floating in a person's bloodstream was primarily a very rough measurement of one's thyroid activity. A high level of blood cholesterol showed the doctor that his patient's thyroid gland was not functioning as well as it should. At the same time, the test was more of a confirmatory procedure; the doctor could usually see that his patient was greatly overweight, had dry skin, a loss of hair (especially in the outer part of the eyebrows), and could not stand cold weather—all of which are only a few of the many signs of myxedema or hypothyroidism. Frequently the physical signs of hypothyroidism went along with the patient's complaint of impotence or menstrual irregularity.

In contrast, a low level of cholesterol usually substantiated the doctor's diagnostic impression that his patient's thyroid gland was too active; a conclusion any doctor would easily surmise if his patient was underweight (especially while eating excessively), had moist hands, was peculiarly nervous, complained of unexplainable diarrhea, and disliked warm weather. And frankly, those signs of hyperthyroidism, including the low blood cholesterol level, were considered far more of a danger to a patient's heart than any amount of fat he might eat.

A person's blood cholesterol may go way up if he or she has kidney disease (because the kidney cannot filter out the large sized lipoprotein molecules such as cholesterol); gallstones (or any other condition that stops the flow of bile, which contains large amounts of cholesterol, from coming out of the gall bladder and into the bowel); trouble with the pancreas (whether from diabetes, too much alcohol, or any infection of this organ); any inherited inability to break down sugar in the body; low blood proteins (usually from a low-protein diet); myeloma (a form of cancer of certain bone cells); and pregnancy—certainly not a "disease."

An infection by a fat-containing virus has also been shown to raise the blood cholesterol level. And, an individual might be born with the genetic factor that automatically causes him to have a high blood cholesterol. People with type A blood normally have significantly higher blood cholesterol levels than those with other blood types (B, AB, and O). Some researchers claim that elevated blood cholesterol associated with type A blood may be the most common cause of hypercholesteremia. Checking back into the family history will inevitably show that one or more members of past generations had hypercholesteremia and that it was not necessarily related to any form of heart disease in one's ancestors. In a study of 500 patients who had high cholesterol levels, nearly half of the immediate family members had a similar genetic circumstance, without any sign of heart disease.

Should a person have liver disease (within the liver itself, as opposed to the blockage of bile by a gallstone) the blood cholesterol as measured by a laboratory test will be much lower. Malnutrition, many anemias, infections, and a great number of drugs and chemicals will cause a lowered cholesterol level—but this certainly does not mean that the individual has no heart disease.

That high or low blood cholesterol levels mean possible or no heart disease, then, is applying an unreliable indicator to a supposed specific body disorder when, in fact, the test could well mean a wide variety of clinical conditions—from normality, to a disease state not even remotely related to the heart. And again, the measurement of blood cholesterol is only a measure of cholesterol floating in the bloodstream at the time the blood is taken; it has nothing to do with the amount of cholesterol that may be implanted within the body itself.

Looking even more closely at this laboratory test that has become anathema to many, it is a fairly simple one that requires no special training to perform and can be completed in any physician's office in a few moments. Briefly, all that is done is to take some blood serum or plasma (that part of the blood that remains after the blood cells are removed) and mix it with some alcohol and ether in order to cause the fat-like substance (in this case, cholesterol) to be extracted. Then a special chemical is added to the extracted material which causes a color change in proportion to the amount of cholesterol present. By comparing the color of the chemically treated serum from the blood against a standard color (that contains a known amount of cholesterol), it is possible to determine how much cholesterol was present in the blood at the moment that particular blood specimen was taken.

Repeated surveys have shown that not only can the moment the blood is taken from a patient make a tremendous difference in the result obtained, but that there are a great many other things not directly related to any disease that can markedly alter the laboratory result. While it is known that regular exercise, along with weight stability, does lower cholesterol levels, exercise itself can actually raise one's cholesterol level—if the blood is tested within a few hours of the exercising. One physician reported that, after running 10 miles each day, his cholesterol level always went up 100 more than usual. Twelve hours after exercising, however, it regularly returned to its lower value.

It is not unusual or abnormal for blood cholesterol to be affected by eating foods including polyunsaturates, but this alteration does not necessarily affect the heart. Everyone's blood sugar goes up after eating carbohydrates (bread, candy, cake, potatoes, alcohol) but the temporarily elevated blood sugar does not mean that everyone has diabetes. It is quite normal for a multitude of body chemicals to increase following an ordinary meal. Therefore, a cholesterol test performed without the patient having fasted for 14 hours would give a false value. Temporary elevations of cholesterol, as with sugar, cannot be considered as being suggestive of any disease.

Some other factors that can influence the end-result of a cholesterol test—factors that a patient would never consider—are how soon after the blood is taken the test is performed; how carefully the blood and chemical measurements are made; how fresh the test chemicals are; how often and how carefully the test-measuring equipment is calibrated; and, most of all, how precise the technician is in reading the color comparison. Most physicians automatically accept the fact that a numerical error of 15 percent either up or down is well within the normal range of what might be expected from this test. Translated, this could mean that someone with a reported blood cholesterol level of 350 —which some physicians would consider abnormally high—

could really be less than 300, an amount that would not neces-sarily be considered as any indication of potential heart problems. Another factor to contemplate is that the reported amount of cholesterol is based on projecting a few drops of blood serum (about 2 ml. or one-fifteenth of an ounce) to 100 ml. (or three and one-third ounces). In other words, the actual amount of choles-terol measured is always then multiplied by 50 in order to arrive at the final figure. Thus the tiniest error in technique will be magnified 50 times greater than what really exists.

That laboratory testing is not as precise as most patients think can be shown by a recent survey conducted by the federal government's Center for Disease Control. Depending on the test being performed, the chances of any significant error runs to about 25 percent of the work. Or, if the government's survey is right, one out of every four tests may come back to the doctor with a grossly erroneous numerical value.

Supposing though that everything is technically perfect, and the laboratory technician is as meticulous as is possible; how does the cholesterol value arrived at compare with what is con-sidered normal? For, in order to derive any medical conclusions from this laboratory test, there must be an accepted standard against which to measure. Experience has shown that there is a well-defined, fairly narrow range for a "normal" blood sugar. The "normal" for some other tests such as hemoglobin, uric acid, and certain minerals is even more precise. Furthermore, these ac-cepted values do not change that much with the age of the indi-vidual. But when it comes to interpreting the amount of cholesterol in a person's blood, there is an extreme discrepancy in so-called "normal" values that are directly related to age. What is called "normal" for a man who is 30 years of age does not even approximate a so-called reassuring value in a man who is 50. The difference can run to 220 (*e.g.,* the presently accepted "normal" for someone under 30 is anywhere from 120 to 290, while it runs from 150 to 340 in a person over 40 years of age). Thus a matter of 11 years in one's age could conceivably make quite an impact on one's life-style depending on the doctor's interpretation of cholesterol values and whether or not he took the age factor into account.

If nothing else, today's assigned "normal" cholesterol val-ues certainly show the wide latitude allowed in interpreting this particular test. And, as if age were not enough, one's national heritage is a most crucial element in deciding if the blood cholesterol is up or down. People of southern European descent seem to have a much higher cholesterol at all times in their lives than do those with an oriental background. Those who have Scandinavian lineage would "normally" be expected to have a higher cholesterol value without really indicating any abnormality of the heart. Those with a black racial background have a much lower typical cholesterol level than do whites, and this in spite of the fact that they may eat a far, far greater amount of saturated fats in their diet.

Can there be any doubt, then, that the particular test to measure blood cholesterol is, in point of fact, an extremely variable measure of a particular blood chemical? To categorize an individual's health on the basis of this laboratory test, then, is patently unfair—as well as without any legitimate scientific basis. As a matter of fact, if the test is to be used at all, it should be taken several times, over many weeks, and with every known technique to reduce the usual stress situation that comes from taking one's blood. And then, once some sort of "average" amount of cholesterol in the blood is inferred, this measurement must be evaluated in the light of many other parameters that are much more accurate in the determination of heart troubles (*e.g.,* electrocardiograph—especially under stress testing; repeated serum uric acid measurements in the blood; various serum enzymes—which are not usually elevated in angina; and, of course, special x-rays to show the true circulation of the arteries of the heart muscle). X-rays have already shown that patients usually do not complain of symptoms until at least 85 percent of the circulation is blocked.

It is a known fact in medicine that if a doctor takes a patient's blood pressure at the onset of a physical examination, the blood pressure reading at that particular time may well be 50 points higher than it would be at the conclusion of the examination. If the blood pressure is measured two or three times during the examination and the doctor does not indicate in any way that something might be wrong, what would seem to be an abnormally high pressure initially will quite likely end up well within the normal range—assuming, of course, that the patient really does not suffer from true hypertension. The apprehension of having one's blood pressure taken, and the imagined dire prognostications that a high reading implies, have repeatedly been shown to cause a false high blood pressure reading: false in the sense that there is no physical underlying disease process directly affecting the blood vessels or kidneys, but not false in the sense that the individual is easily made anxious by any mental stress which, through the brain response, causes a temporary stress hypertension. Most physicians are well aware of this virtually routine phenomenon and if a high first reading is observed, they almost automatically take their patient's blood pressure several times during the course of a physical examination—striving to relieve the patient's stress and put him as much at ease as is possible under the circumstances.

As has been mentioned, there are many medical reports that show that cholesterol levels, like blood pressure levels, are temporarily raised, sometimes to a great degree, as a result of a stressful situation. Dr. Meyer Friedman, of San Francisco, who has described the personality characteristics of the man who has difficulty handling stressful situations, calls this sudden rise a "neurogenic hypercholesteremia." That is, the cholesterol goes up in response to the mind's reaction to some emotional situation. The rise has no relationship to diet, let alone to the particular type of fat eaten.

Soldiers have shown elevated cholesterol levels when they are required to perform any potentially dangerous mission. And, to confirm the physiological mechanism behind this non-dietary rise in cholesterol, an electrical stimulation in the area of the brain that perceives emotional stimuli also causes an elevated cholesterol level. As Dr. Friedman says: "Too often high cholesterol levels are blamed on diet, rather than on behavior patterns."

Dr. Kenneth Rose of the University of Nebraska has shown that by subjecting animals to stress he can routinely cause an increase in blood cholesterol levels.

Then, there was an Air Force study that showed how anger and frustration could cause a marked increase in blood cholesterol levels that lasted for years without causing any heart disease whatsoever. Emotional stress and the exhaustion of the adrenal hormones that initially cause the cholesterol rise were considered more a causative factor for any ultimate disease than diet.

In one series of experiments, medical students were tested

weekly to determine a reasonable base line for their cholesterol values. Then, immediately after a school examination was announced, their cholesterol was tested. The students' blood cholesterol levels rose more than twice as high. The cholesterol levels of accountants have been shown to be way, way up around tax time—when these men are under pressure to complete their work before a deadline.

The relationship between stress and misleading blood pressure readings must be applied to cholesterol determinations. So must all the other factors that can momentarily alter the laboratory determination of this still unsubstantiated indication of heart disease. In point of fact, we really do not know what a "normal" cholesterol level is at this time. All we really have is a laboratory test in search of a disease; a test that seems to be creating more havoc than good health.

The level of one's blood cholesterol is, at best, nothing more than an extremely rough indication of a great many different disease conditions. At worst, it can be more the cause of stress and the diseases that stress brings on. To alter one's life style as a consequence of this particular laboratory test may well cause more trouble than it could relieve.

But the story does not end there. For, although the test for blood cholesterol has been promoted as *the* definitive indicator of heart disease, it should not surprise anyone to know that this laboratory measurement alone would not stand the test of time where more definitive tests can be devised. Researchers have since come up with an entire battery of tests for the many, various lipids (fats) that travel in the blood. Cholesterol, itself, is really a mixture of different lipoproteins (fat molecules attached to protein molecules), and now it seems more precise to test specifically for these different forms of fat. You may have heard, or you will be hearing, that you are now being tested for the amounts of lipoproteins in your blood. Or, you may be told you are being tested to see if you have hyperlipidemia (or hyperlipoproteinemia). Translated this means your blood has been tested to measure the levels of cholesterol, along with the levels of triglycerides and phospholipids. Triglycerides are the neutral fats you absorb from your intestine and which are eventually stored in your body as the fatty layers under the skin to supply energy when needed. The phospholipids are simply another form of fat that contains phosphoric acid. The three fats are sometimes called chylomicrons which are absorbed in the blood after eating. These classifications may help to decide whether the fats in your blood are primary, that is are there directly, or secondary, meaning they are there subsequent to some other existing disease process.

Although some doctors still rely on the cholesterol blood test alone (and, unfortunately, without regard to stress, time of day, etc.), most sophisticated physicians have added the test for blood (serum) triglycerides and feel that without the combination of the two tests, no clinical significance can be applied to the cholesterol measurement. If one's cholesterol *and* triglyceride tests are within "normal", all that it means is that there is no indication of hyperlipidemia. The reported results of the two-test combination, in addition to observation of blood plasma in a test tube after it has been refrigerated for a day—along with the patient's family history may give a diagnostic categorization number that says one of five types of hyperlipidemia is present. Of course, the same profile might also mean diabetes, an infection in the pancreas, a blood disease, a metabolic disorder (thyroid trouble being one example), kidney disease, cancer, alcoholism or pregnancy. So, in essence, we are really right back where we started, without any definitive evidence of heart disease.

Such elaborate blood tests, should they be reported as abnormal, are then followed up with a confirmatory test called paper electrophoresis. This is where a drop of plasma (serum) is put on a piece of paper and charged with an electrical current to see which sized fat particles migrate the fastest and farthest causing visible bands or layers of fats to show a specific pattern on the paper. And again, what you end up with is a number classification of the type of hyperlipidemia.

Theoretically, the type of hyperlipidemia is the clue to the type of treatment you will need, especially in regard to the drugs your physician may prescribe. For, it seems that a particular drug will lower cholesterol in one type of hyperlipidemia while that same drug has no evident effect on another type. So now that you know your type of hyperlipidemia, thanks to the most intricate laboratory procedures, you might start taking some medicine to alter the fat levels found in your blood. When you do, you must keep in mind the warning that every drug manufacturer is legally *required* to give every physician (but not the patient who takes the drug) concerning use of the product for lowering cholesterol:

> An important note: It has not been established whether drug-induced lowering of serum cholesterol or other lipid levels has a detrimental, a beneficial, or no effect on the morbidity or mortality due to atherosclerosis or coronary heart disease. Several years will be required before current investigations can yield an answer to this question.

In other words, even if you have an elevated blood cholesterol level, and even if you do something that is supposed to reduce your cholesterol level, no one, not even your doctor, knows for sure if lowering your cholesterol will have *any* effect in warding off heart disease. Moreso, no one knows if lowering your cholesterol might, in fact, be more harmful than leaving it alone!

If you have been told that your blood cholesterol is "too high," what does it really mean? How many times were you tested for the amount of this fat-like substance? How soon after eating were you tested? How apprehensive were you at the time you were tested? Did you feel, when you were tested, that the result of the test might show you had hidden heart disease? Moreso, did you feel that the results of the test might well force you to change your way of life? If you were fearful, how much of that fear was generated by commercialism—advertising, publicity etc.—as opposed to your doctor's own attitude?

Cholesterol has become an American phobia causing many people, especially men to live in terror of knowing how much of it is in their blood, and once knowing, intimating a drastic reduction in their odds against an early death. But on what scientific basis? To understand how the association came about, it is necessary to understand what cholesterol is, how it gets into the body, and what it does in the body once it is there. But, this too is still hypothetical, and there is no proof that an elevated blood cholesterol is the cause of any heart disease.

CHAPTER *3*

ALL ABOUT CHOLESTEROL

IT IS A fact that when people have advanced atherosclerosis (or arteriosclerosis, as it is sometimes called), and they have some atheromatous plaques (fatty-looking, grayish-yellow patches) in the walls or linings of some of their arteries, these plaques do have some cholesterol in them. It was this observation that led to the hypothesis that cholesterol might be the culprit in heart and artery disease. But it is now known that these same plaques also contain several other substances such as triglycerides, phospholipids, fibrin (a protein needed for normal blood clotting, sometimes called "nature's glue"), collagen (another protein that forms the support, or matrix for all our tissues such as skin, muscles and bones), certain minerals that cause "hardening," and an abundance of special cells that hold the various fatty products. And, there are many pathologists who firmly believe that the blood fibrin, forming a "scab" inside the artery, is more the real reason behind heart and artery disease than are any of the blood fats. As a matter of fact, cholesterol is *not* even a part of the early atheromatous plaque formation, which is where the trouble really begins.

Depending on a person's age, atherosclerosis may be more "normal" than unusual. As a result of careful autopsy studies, it would be the exception to the rule if atheromatous plaques were *not* found, to some degree, once a person has reached middle-age. Atherosclerosis has been found in infants only a few days old, and has also been found to a great degree in soldiers in their late teens and early twenties who have been exposed to the stress of battle. Even young athletes who are in top physical condition have been found to have more atherosclerosis than some men in their sixties or seventies. But the amount of atherosclerosis found in the body is not necessarily correlated to heart or artery disease. It certainly has not been scientifically related to the amount of cholesterol a person eats.

Of course, it would be unfair not to mention that there have been some medical reports to indicate that where certain patients have markedly elevated levels of blood cholesterol, they also seem to have had a greater incidence of heart disease. But at the same time, just as there were those in the Framingham study who had high blood cholesterol levels and who also had heart disease, there were as many who died of heart attacks who had low blood cholesterol levels. And there have been other studies of specific populations as widespread as in England, New York City and Seattle, Washington, that show *no* significant association between cholesterol levels and heart disease.

One important distinction that is rarely made by those who attempt to link cholesterol levels in the blood to heart disease is whether or not the person has had some previous clinical evidence of heart disease. For it does seem that elevated cholesterol levels are more likely to come after the fact, rather than before. That is, once a person has definite outward signs of heart disease, he may well show an elevated cholesterol level in the blood. Whether this is related to the existing heart disease, or is a consequence of some other, possibly non-related functional breakdown, cannot be proved at this time. It has been shown, however, that reducing the cholesterol level in such a patient does *not* prevent further heart trouble. In fact, some studies show that in those patients whose cholesterol was lowered, there was a greater subsequent incidence of heart attacks.

What all this really means is that we do not know whether there is any truly scientific relationship between a blood cholesterol level and the possibility of having a heart attack. And, as one develops more deeply into the studies that attempt to show some correlation between heart troubles and the amount of cholesterol in the blood, one learns that a number of other factors come into play. These are anxiety or stress, physical fitness, high blood pressure, being overweight, smoking, blood uric acid levels, age, heredity, and whether you are male or female. Since elevated cholesterol levels seem to be found more often in people who have already *had* heart trouble, there are a great many physicians and researchers who still ponder the question as to which came first—the heart trouble or the elevated cholesterol.

As a matter of fact, the entire concept upon which the present cholesterol controversy is based is unique and totally opposed to all previously accepted scientific thinking. That is, the explanation now being offered by those who do believe that excessive cholesterol in the blood is deposited *on* the walls of arteries, runs counter to today's knowledge of classical pathology. To justify the excessive cholesterol-in-the-blood answer to heart disease would require an entirely new approach to the cause of almost all disease. Briefly, those who condemn high levels of cholesterol in the blood believe that this cholesterol can deposit itself on the artery wall and then filter *through* that artery wall to form its plaque. This phenomenon has still never actually been demonstrated, even as a possibility. What we do know, however, is that atheromatous plaques form wherever there has been physical wear and tear on the artery wall and where fibrin (a normal component of blood necessary for clotting) grows *inside* of the artery wall, narrowing the artery passageway and eventually blocking off the blood flow. Furthermore, it causes a secondary fibrin (and possibly platelet) clot inside the blood vessel passageway, and this clot is what really stops the flow of oxygen-carrying blood altogether.

But, because of all the publicity given to cholesterol, it seems only right to understand this substance. Where does it come from? How is it made? What does it normally do? And, just how necessary is it to the body? After all, Americans are literally being brainwashed to eat as little cholesterol as possible and, in addition, to eat certain foods (and take certain drugs) supposedly to reduce their blood cholesterol as it is measured by some laboratory test. What might happen if people did, in fact, follow the rules now set forth by some food manufacturers, the American Heart Association and writers of books and articles advocating low cholesterol diets?

Even if you were to avoid every speck of cholesterol you could in your diet, your body would still manufacturer cholesterol at a fairly steady rate and in a relatively profuse amount. In fact, it has been shown repeatedly that the less cholesterol a person eats, the more the body itself produces. And, by avoiding cholesterol in your diet to an extreme, you may well end up with far more cholesterol in your blood than would be there normally. But should you still eat cholesterol, it has been shown that the average person's body will rid itself of just about the same amount of cholesterol as that eaten, no matter what the laboratory blood cholesterol test shows.

When you eat any food containing cholesterol, the cholesterol must first go through the intestinal wall in order to enter the bloodstream. Surprisingly, the intestine has a very limited capacity to absorb the cholesterol you eat. In this way your body actually protects you from taking in too much by way of your diet. If you do happen to eat a great deal of food containing cholesterol, most of it will simply pass through your bowel and be eliminated.

What little cholesterol that does enter your blood from your intestinal tract, goes directly to your liver where it joins the cholesterol that your liver automatically, and normally manufactures. And this liver-made cholesterol is no different from the kind you eat. If you do absorb some cholesterol, and your liver happens to be making its own cholesterol at the same time, the excess amount—whatever your body determines is more than you actually need at the moment—will be excreted in your bile, and it, too, will go through your bowel and be eliminated. Other organs and tissues of your body such as muscle and skin can also manufacture cholesterol as needed. And if, for some reason, you do not eat enough cholesterol, even your intestinal wall will synthesize this chemical to meet any immediate demands. Throughout all of your life your body automatically keeps the amount of cholesterol you take in and the amount of cholesterol you excrete just about equal. If you eat too much, you are protected from absorbing too much; if your body makes a little too much, it automatically gets rid of any excess.

In a fascinating experiment, one group of animals was fed an unlimited amount of cholesterol from birth while a second group was deprived of any cholesterol in its early diet. After several years, it was found that the animals who ate the cholesterol manufactured very little through the usual body processes.

In contrast, the animals who were deprived of dietary cholesterol manufactured a great deal more than would have been necessary and were constantly forced to eliminate the excess cholesterol. In other words, if the body receives a reasonable amount of cholesterol in the diet, it is not forced to manufacture as much of this product—which it will do regardless of any heart disease. To deliberately deprive yourself of foods that contain cholesterol, then, could cause your body to make a great deal more than is needed. If your blood cholesterol happened to be measured at a moment when your body needed an excess of this chemical compound, you could have come up with abnormally high level of cholesterol that had no real meaning insofar as your heart was concerned.

The fact that your body does make its own cholesterol is more valuable than you might imagine. Cholesterol is absolutely essential in order for your nerves to transmit their impulses throughout your body, as well as from and to your brain. Your nervous system could not work without an adequate amount of cholesterol to act as a conductor. In addition to nerve impulse transmission, the body must have cholesterol in order to make sex hormones—of which cholesterol is an integral part.

Then, in light of the recent polyunsaturate advertising that proposes that everyone, even from birth, alter his diet supposedly in order to keep cholesterol levels low, keep in mind the statement of Dr. Peter O. Kwiterovich, a pediatrician at Johns Hopkins University School of Medicine, who says: "No one really knows how brain growth would be affected if a child were to receive a strict low cholesterol diet before he is 24 months of age, at which point 95 percent of brain growth is completed." Is possible early brain damage preferable to some unproved future protection against heart disease?

And, speaking of babies, it has been proposed that mother's milk (breast feeding) contains "too much" cholesterol. Two Princeton physicians have claimed that mother's milk may cause arteriosclerosis. To quote Dr. Mark D. Altschule, professor of medicine at Harvard University Medical College: "The picture this presents of mothers giving their helpless babies arteriosclerosis while pretending to satisfy their craving for the breast and its contents is almost too horrible to contemplate. Horrible or not, it has the useful effect of lending strong support for the theoretical notion popularized by recent sociopsychologic writings that everything an American mother might (or might not) do is bound to affect her offspring adversely."

So far, the one particular fatty substance that has been discussed is cholesterol, since that has become a household word almost routinely associated with such dire consequences. If we heed all of the advertising and publicity, we are almost forced to consider cholesterol every time we sit down to a meal. But there are many other laboratory tests for many different kinds of related fats in the blood that should be noted. Although, at the moment, there is no certainty about the clinical meaning of any blood-fat measurement, be it cholesterol, the triglycerides, the beta-lipoproteins (sometimes called low-density lipoproteins), the very-low-density lipoproteins, the high density lipoproteins, chylomicrons, or simply, the free fatty acids. In fact, cholesterol and triglycerides are really mixtures of the various lipoproteins and the only significance of the term is to categorize a person with a high laboratory-measured cholesterol level into five different research-study groups—rare, familial, possibly metabolic, or possibly associated with either alcoholism or diabetes. But they all amount to the same thing: hyperlipidemia, or an increased, supposedly abnormal, amount of fat floating around in the blood as determined by some laboratory test.

And even with all this highly technical knowledge at our command, one of the men who detected and elaborated on the many different kinds of fats that could be measured in the blood, Dr. Robert I. Levy, chief of the National Heart and Lung Institute's Lipid Metabolism Branch, has recently stated: "We have not yet proved that decreasing dietary cholesterol or lowering serum cholesterol levels will decrease the risk of heart disease. It remains to be established that a diet high in polyunsaturated fats is a better and *safer* diet than most Americans consume today."

We really do not know what it means—insofar as heart disease is concerned—if your cholesterol is supposedly high. We know even less what will happen if we lower it by diet or drugs, which while temporarily possible, is not really easy to maintain, with the body's automatic reaction to the amount of cholesterol eaten or synthesized.

Bowes and Church, whose book *Food Values of Portions Commonly Used* is considered by most physicians and nutritionists as an authoritative reference, have no hesitation in stating: "The relationship of dietary cholesterol to total cholesterol in the body and to atherogenesis continues to be a subject for debate." They point out that no matter how much you reduce the cholesterol in the diet, the body will still synthesize its own cholesterol in abundance from non-cholesterol containing foods.

Recent research reported by a University of Minnesota physician cites the fact that when blood cholesterol is reduced— in this instance, by eating an excessive amount of corn oil—there is an accompanying *increase* in the cholesterol content of the heart, liver and other body organs. The article then goes on to say: "These results pose the question whether a change in serum or tissue cholesterol concentration may be regarded as beneficial." If one does lower the cholesterol level in the blood, does that cholesterol deposit itself in the body—and could this deposit be more harmful than helpful?

Furthermore, according to a five year study of some 8,000 coronary heart disease patients, conducted at the Veteran's Administration Hospital in Ann Arbor by Dr. Henry K. Schoch, associate professor of medicine at the University of Michigan, the lowering of blood cholesterol seems to offer *no* protection once a patient has suffered a heart attack. Dr. Schoch says: "The results of the present study do seem to suggest that serum cholesterol values may well not be a significant indicator of survival or of future morbidity, once the disease has become manifest, compared to other factors (such as possibly the development of collateral circulation, the residual myocardial reserve, or the resultant electrical excitability of the myocardium)."

Dr. Paul Dudley White, considered by many to be America's leading heart specialist, now says: "I think I have a pretty clear idea of the role of proteins, carbohydrates and so forth, but I must admit I'm thoroughly confused about cholesterol and, for that matter, I'm not sure whether some form of the weight-control diets might not be dangerous to the heart. The amount in the blood—we call it serum cholesterol, is not necessarily related to cholesterol found in food."

If Dr. White admits *he* is confused about cholesterol, and that the amount of cholesterol one eats is not really the culprit it has been claimed to be, then you, as a layman, should not feel badly that you do not understand all there is to know about this particular "steroid" compound (sometimes referred to as a sterol). Cholesterol is one of a group of chemicals that have a fat-like, solid alcohol structure. Some similar body chemicals would include certain hormones and vitamin D.

We do know that should you happen to eat a food that contains a lot of cholesterol, then the body normally responds by slowing down its own production and automatically increasing the rate of cholesterol excretion. But what is "a lot" of cholesterol? No one really knows. Surveys indicate that the "average" American eating a "typical" American diet with no fat restrictions, takes in about 600 mg., or one-sixtieth of an ounce of cholesterol a day. Further testing has shown that for each 100 mg. of cholesterol you do not eat, you *might* lower the blood cholesterol measurements by three to five mg. percent. Consider this amount of blood cholesterol lowering against a test that can quite normally be off as much as 50 mg. percent because ordinary testing techniques may encompass an overall normal variable range of 200 mg. percent and still be within normal limits. As already mentioned, the cholesterol measurement may also be altered by 200 or more through your anxiety, the drugs you have taken, or some other body dysfunction not at all related to the heart. Thus, if you were to adhere strictly to the American Heart Association's dietary recommendation of keeping your cholesterol intake to less than 300 mg. a day, you might lower your blood cholesterol by 10—far less than the accepted range of error for the test itself. Then, if you do reduce the amount of cholesterol you eat, you are also signaling your body to manufacture more cholesterol on its own.

Yet you are constantly being told to eat foods with little or no cholesterol. A good example is the "advice" to avoid dairy foods—with commercial advertising stressing how butter, milk, and cream substitutes are "cholesterol free." How do you explain the paradox of being told not to drink milk because it contains cholesterol, and yet being told to eat more and more fish, which contains at least eight times as much cholesterol, ounce for ounce, as milk?

"Consumers and physicians have become the victims of an unfounded medical dogma," says Dr. Louis H. Nahum, noted cardiologist and professor of medicine at Yale University Medical School. Writing about the cholesterol mystique in the Connecticut State Medical Society journal, of which he is editor, Dr. Nahum admits that many physicians disagree with the cholesterol concept that is publicized to their patients. When the American Heart Association, margarine manufacturers and certain governmental health divisions tell the American people that cholesterol is bad, the physician who questions this edict—asking for some sort of proof—is considered out-of-step.

To summarize, the body must have cholesterol in order to function properly and to manufacture vital hormones and chemicals. To deprive the body of cholesterol simply causes it to make that much more. And, when the body is forced to make its own cholesterol, as opposed to obtaining it via food, this could be more the cause of certain diseases (*e.g.*, gallstones) than it could be a cure for heart troubles. Yes, it is possible to look back on some people with heart attacks and say they had "elevated" blood cholesterol levels, but the same studies show that at least as many people, if not more, who have had heart attacks had "normal" blood cholesterol levels prior to their heart disease. There is, at this time, insufficient scientific evidence to implicate a laboratory-measured blood cholesterol level with impending heart disease. There are, however, more than enough warning signs to show that a purposeful attempt to reduce the amount of cholesterol in the body might well lead to more bodily harm than good.

PART **II**

WHAT ARE THE ISSUES?

ALTHOUGH THE PRIMARY purpose of this book is to relieve some of the worry and aggravation that has been imposed on the public by the insistence that cholesterol is *the* cause of heart disease and heart attacks, there will still be those who blindly accept the diet-heart disease hypothesis and who will do anything to bring down their cholesterol levels. Surprisingly, any drastic attempt to lower one's cholesterol through commercially proposed methods may cause more harm than good. The public and private agencies that could and should offer the public proper health information and protection in such matters seem totally reluctant to do their jobs. When professional groups, such as the American Heart Association, make public statements or take public actions that cannot be scientifically supported, in the long run they weaken their credibility. When government agencies do the same, or fail to right a wrong, the matter is even worse. When business preys on the public's fear of heart disease for its own profit, the only protection the consumer can have is knowledge.

CHAPTER **4**

THE UNPUBLICIZED SIDE OF THE
CHOLESTEROL CONTROVERSY

THE GREATEST OF all myths behind the cholesterol controversy is the hypothesis that if, primarily through changing the
kind of fat one eats, one does reduce the amount of cholesterol
in one's blood (as measured by certain laboratory tests), the risk
of having heart disease—and especially a heart attack—will also
be reduced. The measurable level of cholesterol floating in one's
blood has, in fact, been labeled as a "risk" factor involved in heart
and artery disease. But, after several decades of promoting this
legend, not one whit of truly scientific evidence has been produced to prove this hypothesis—and that is all it still is.

The most recent "official" pronouncement has come from
the National Heart and Lung Institute Task Force on Arteriosclerosis. This federal government supported group of physicians,
considered experts in the field of heart disease, said in 1972, that
the use of diet (specifically an increase in polyunsaturated fats
and a decrease in saturated fats solely for the purpose of lowering
blood cholesterol levels) is scientifically *not* convincing. The report even went on to say that any recommendations concerning
diet in relation to heart and artery disease are strictly "intuitive"
and are based only on personal impressions and fragmentary
conclusions rather than on scientific proof.

But in spite of the fact that there is no scientific proof to
back up the concept that polyunsaturates will consistently and
effectively lower one's blood cholesterol level and through this

method heart attacks will be prevented, the American public is being made more and more subject to a promotion and publicity campaign that is bent on altering the American diet to stress those polyunsaturated fats at the expense of meat, dairy foods and eggs.

To be sure, there are some studies that could, if the publicized results are accepted without question, indicate a basis for this contention. There are some people with "high" cholesterol levels who die from heart attacks. There are some people who eat a great deal of fat who die from heart attacks. But this sort of association is meaningless unless all aspects (*e.g.,* heredity, stress, physical fitness, smoking, high blood pressure, other disease conditions) of the individual and his way of life are taken into account.

It is the other side of the story—studies where people eat a great deal of fat, especially saturated fat, and who have very little heart disease—that has rarely been offered to the public. As a simple example, how many Americans have heard about the Pennsylvania community of Roseto where the residents have less than half as many deaths from heart attacks as do the residents of surrounding cities—and far less than the United States as a whole? This observation was not the consequence of a momentary glance at the death rate of this one town; it was a conclusion drawn after an eleven-year study. Not only do the people of Roseto eat a great many foods fried in lard (an almost totally saturated fat extremely high in cholesterol), they also eat their prosciutto ham with a rim of saturated, cholesterol containing, fat more than an inch thick. Their most frequently eaten dish is fried peppers, with most people dipping bread into the lard gravy to savor every last drop of the flavor.

Naturally, the first question that comes to mind is what was the blood cholesterol level of these people who eat foods containing so much saturated fat and cholesterol (and where the men drink at least 8 percent of their calories as wine)? For these men, the blood cholesterol went from a low of 136 to more than 500, with the average being 224. The women's cholesterol levels were almost identical. These cholesterol values correspond to those reported in the "Framingham Study," and may be considered as quite "average." Certainly if blood cholesterol levels and diet are as reliable indicators of heart disease as is so forcefully publicized, the heart attack deaths in Roseto, Pennsylvania, should at least come close to the ominous statistics being instilled in the public's mind. But they do not. In fact, during the eleven-year period studied, there was a virtual absence of heart attacks in Roseto men under the age of 55. And, of those over 65 who did show some evidence of heart disease, there was a relatively high rate of survival.

For every report of a group of people who supposedly have a high risk of heart disease because they eat a great many high cholesterol foods and saturated fats, and ostensibly have a high blood cholesterol as a result, there is always another group of people who eat the same things and have very little heart disease and, in most instances, "normal" blood cholesterol levels.

Starting in Africa, there are the Somali camel herdmen whose diet includes five quarts of camel's milk each day. The highest blood cholesterol level found in these men was 153. No form of heart disease was found. The Masai of Tanganyika who are extremely heavy meat eaters and milk drinkers (and the fat content of their milk is twice what it is in the United States) have an average blood cholesterol level of 125. Heart disease is almost non-existent, and those who die accidentally over the age of 65 show almost no evidence of atherosclerosis.

In the Cook Islands, one group of Polynesians who eat 12 times as much saturated fat as their neighbors show no difference in heart attacks, which are extremely low in both populations. In the Punjab section of India, a group of men whose diet was extremely high in saturated fat was studied. The average blood cholesterol level for these men was 186—much, much lower than that of the average American who normally eats less than half as much saturated fat as the men in this study. Those who made the study frankly admitted that low blood cholesterol, therefore, could not be attributed solely to a diet high in polyunsaturates.

In a three-year study of people in Switzerland, it was discovered that Swiss mountain people who consume a large amount of saturated fats in their diets show a low serum cholesterol level. These rural residents were then compared with people who live in a nearby urban area, who have much higher cholesterol levels; it was found that the mountain folk not only eat more foods with saturated fats, they also eat far more cholesterol containing-foods. They regularly drink 50 percent more milk, eat four times as much cheese, three times as much lard, use twice as much shortening and about half as much margarine and oil in cooking as do their city counterparts. At age 40, the average cholesterol level of those who live in the rural area was about one-third of that of those in the neighboring urban part of Switzerland; the latter's cholesterol level paralleled that found in the United States even though Americans eat less saturated fats.

When the diets of men in Ireland were compared to the diets of Irish men in Boston, Massachusetts, it was found that although the native Irish ate 16 percent more animal fats and 10 percent more saturated fats, they still had *lower* cholesterol values. Furthermore, no difference in heart attack deaths were found in the two groups of men, leading the doctors who made this study to say that in the light of their findings: "it is unlikely that any 'abnormality' in dietary intake accounts, in isolation, for the appearance of coronary heart disease, at least in male patients under 60 years of age."

Dr. Harold A. Kahn, of the National Heart and Lung Institute, has made his own study to determine if the widely publicized theory that cholesterol causes heart attacks, has any true basis in fact. He concluded that over the past 60 years the amount of cholesterol that is eaten has not changed, although the amount of polyunsaturates in the diet has greatly increased. During the same period, the heart attack rate has skyrocketed, leading Dr. Kahn to say: "The increased rate of coronary heart disease reported to have occurred over this period is not related to dietary fat changes to a very important degree."

Dr. George V. Mann, professor of biochemistry and medicine at Vanderbilt University is even more definitive—and he is the doctor who was responsible for the evaluation of the dietary portion of the "Framingham Study". Dr. Mann calls the entire concept of altering the kinds of fat one eats in order to reduce atherosclerotic disease as being "overpromoted and overpublicized." He goes on to say that "We have not seen any evidence that these diets are effective." Furthermore, Dr. Mann feels that the theory that fatty acids metabolism plays a role in atherosclerosis is a "myth" that "has been a terribly wasteful diversion for the medical community. After 20 years and several hundred million dollars, we still do not see any convincing evidence in its support."

And, Dr. Mann goes much further when he states: "Physicians who have tried diet therapy for hypercholesteremia and coronary heart disease soon find it doesn't work. Diet therapy is indeed an impotent treatment of hypocholesteremia, and no one —but no one—has shown it to be an effective preventive for coronary heart disease."

Doctors Kahn and Mann are not alone in their intense criticism of the promotion of special diets (primarily polyunsaturated fats and reduced cholesterol containing foods). Dr. Richard C. Bozian, professor of medicine at the University of Cincinnati, has written: "Neither proven causal relationship for dietary cholesterol-coronary artery disease nor altered prognosis following hypocholesteremic regimens has been established."

Dr. Stewart Wolf of the University of Texas and Dr. John Bruhn of the University of Oklahoma Medical School analyzed more than 100 medical articles on the relationship of claimed risk factors to heart disease, trying to find some common diet denominator that could honestly be called a "risk factor"—something that could scientifically be claimed to be a cause of heart attacks. They could find no consistent pattern in studies all over the world that would identify the type of fat in one's diet, or the level of cholesterol in one's blood, as having any effect on heart disease. They too, criticized the way the results of the "Framingham Study" were edited and written up for public consumption to give the wrong impression. In reality, the results showed no relationship between what a person eats and his risk of having a heart attack. The "Framingham Study" itself clearly showed: "There is no discernible difference between reported diet intake and serum cholesterol levels." Yet this aspect of the study received little attention in newspapers and magazines that accept margarine and polyunsaturated oil advertising.

Another study given very little publicity outside of the medical profession, was made by Dr. Meyer Friedman of San Francisco. His study demonstrated that it really did not matter what type of fat a person ate. No positive effect on the blood cholesterol level could be measured when the type of fat in the diet was altered to either an extreme of polyunsaturated fats or an extreme of saturated fats. Of even greater significance, when Dr. Friedman measured the clinical effect of the different types of fats on the sludging of red blood cells in humans (sludging causes a decrease in the amount of oxygen being delivered to body tissues), he could find no difference whether he used a saturated or a polyunsaturated fat. He came to the conclusion that, in his own studies, there was absolutely no benefit from using polyunsaturates.

In a study in England, 400 elderly men were divided into two groups with one-half of them given a high polyunsaturated diet to see if this diet would, in fact, reduce the incidence of heart attacks. The conclusion of the research team making the study was that, after more than six years, there was no evidence that heart attacks could be materially affected by the use of polyunsaturated fats in the diet. Those who were on the high polyunsaturate diet took at least three ounces of a polyunsaturated oil each day (half of which—at least six tablespoons—was taken directly) plus polyunsaturated margarine. The subjects were forbidden the use of butter, whole milk, cheese, egg yolks and any saturated fat for cooking. The idea was to supply twice as much polyunsaturates in the diet. The other group on a "usual" diet ate six times as much saturated fat as polyunsaturated fat.

Initially, the cholesterol levels of those on the extreme polyunsaturate diet did come down about ten percent. But, even though the men stayed on the diet, the cholesterol levels started to go back up before the first year had passed, and as the years went on they returned to just about where they were before the study started. At the end of the test period, 27 men on the high polyunsaturate diet died from cardiovascular disease while only 25 men on the high saturated fat diet died from the same condition. And, almost identical conclusions were found in a similar study conducted in Oslo, Norway.

In Finland, the substitution of polyunsaturated fats for saturated fats in the diet of patients in one of two mental hospitals, where diets could be carefully controlled, did not show any significant difference in mortality from heart disease.

There are many more studies that openly conflict with the proposed and widely propagated theory that increased polyunsaturates and/or low cholesterol diets will reduce heart disease. These studies are seemingly ignored or suppressed. Certainly they are not brought to the attention of the American public the way the more commercially profitable theories have been. The big question is then, why is this one theory being promoted when there really is no consistent evidence that altering the type of fat in the diet will lessen the possibility of having a heart attack?

Furthermore, why is so little attention paid to the "side effects" or dangers that seem to prevail when excessive polyunsaturates are made part of the diet? Some are minor; in the study in England, for example, ten of the men who were forced to eat twice the usual quantity of polyunsaturates developed diarrhea. But some of the other side effects seem infinitely more dangerous, and far more frequent than the risk of a heart attack itself. These observations should have been publicized as widely as the commercial entreaties to change the kind of fat one eats, if the advertiser honestly had the consumer's best interests at heart or if the U.S. Food and Drug Administration or the Federal Trade Commission really cared about truth in advertising.

Just as most Americans probably never heard of the study of diet in relation to heart disease in Roseto, Pennsylvania, another very impressive study that received no publicity was conducted by Dr. E. Cuyler Hammond (the epidemiologist and statistician for the American Cancer Society who first related excessive smoking to lung cancer) and Dr. Lawrence Garfinkle (Chief of the Cancer Society's Special Projects). Their reported observations seem to confirm the idea that diet, especially a high polyunsaturated fat diet, may well have nothing whatsoever to do with warding off a heart attack. More than a million people in twenty-five states were studied to see if any particular dietary habit could be identified and connected to heart disease and stroke deaths. The eventual analysis was limited to 804,409 persons who had *no* previous history of heart disease or stroke. After a six-year period, a total of 14,819 persons under study died of heart disease and 4,099 died of stroke.

The records of those who died were divided into two groups for an extremely detailed scrutiny of the diets. The first group consisted of those who ate eggs at least five to seven times a week, and also had a high consumption of such items as meat and fried foods as well as salad oil and mayonnaise (egg) dressing. The second group consisted of subjects who ate no eggs or ate them less than four times a week, and who ate little meat or fried foods. Those in the first group, who did *not* control their intake of cholesterol containing foods and saturated fats, had *fewer* deaths from heart disease and stroke than those who adhered to the supposedly "prudent" diet!

Is the concept behind cholesterol as much of a myth, then, as it is a commercial venture? A great deal of money has already been made as the result of pushing polyunsaturates with the advertised claim that this type of fat will lower one's cholesterol and thereby protect one from heart disease. One particular advertiser, in flagrant violation of existing FDA law, says in his ads that by changing your diet to his particular brand of polyunsaturate you won't "eat your heart out." In another ad for the same company there is an implied promise that eating its specific highly polyunsaturated products will "help fight heart disease." Subsequent to this advertising, the company's profits doubled in 1971 and continued to climb astronomically thereafter.

This brings us to two important areas to consider. First, can an excess of polyunsaturates be even more dangerous than the condition they are supposed to prevent and treat? And second, are we being misled by commercialism to do something that can be extremely harmful?

CHAPTER 5

THE POTENTIAL DANGERS OF THE DIETARY TREATMENT OF HYPERCHOLESTEREMIA

A NINETEEN-YEAR OLD boy was brought to a Detroit hospital emergency room following the sudden onset of severe stomach pain. When no specific diagnosis could be made after 24 hours, the boy was operated upon and the exploratory surgery showed that his spleen was twice its normal size, ruptured and bleeding. (The spleen is an organ in the left upper part of the abdomen that helps control the amount of blood in the body, and makes certain blood cells as well as some antibodies that help fight disease.) A detailed post-operative study to determine the cause of the ruptured spleen came up with only one logical precipitating factor; the boy had been on an extremely high diet of polyunsaturates —the particular food ingredient being so vociferously recommended as a preventive and cure for heart disease.

As a matter of fact this boy had been eating a tremendous quantity of polyunsaturates since infancy, including soy bean milk which is almost 90 percent polyunsaturated. Corn oil and cottonseed oil along with soy and wheat protein made up the bulk of the boy's daily diet. And what pathologists found in the spleen was a profusion of ceroid bodies—sometimes called aging pigments—that are known to increase in the body as one grows older; they are, in fact, a fairly reliable indication of aging in humans (much as the rings in a tree trunk show the age of the tree).

Where do ceroids come from? One known source of this

waste-product pigment is from the chemical reaction following the oxidation of polyunsaturated fats. The more polyunsaturates one eats the more the oxidation of these fats occurs. And the end-result of this fat oxidation is the ceroid pigment—sometimes called a "clinker" by pathologists because of its black-brown-burned-cinder-like appearance under the microscope. Oxidation is the same process that causes rust in metal.

While the specific chemical processes that produce ceroid bodies, or age pigments, are quite complicated, it is possible to understand the generalized nature of the action. To begin with, polyunsaturated fatty acids are, in themselves, very unstable compounds. The words "saturated" and "polyunsaturated" are somewhat descriptive. A saturated fat is like a completely closed chemical entity—that is to say, it does not easily react with other chemicals around it because of the fact that it is completely saturated, or contains sufficient chemical parts to make it stable. Unsaturated, on the other hand, means that the compound has some "loose-ends," or susceptible reactive parts still attached to it which will easily combine with another chemical to form a new compound. A *poly*unsaturated fatty acid means that the fat has *many* more reactive parts that make it all the more unstable.

When you strike an ordinary wooden, non-safety match, the unstable portion of the chemicals in that match react with the oxygen in the air to cause a flame. A "safety" match, on the other hand, has less active chemicals that require a special striking surface to make up for its stability. If the match is wet, the potential chemical activity is sufficiently defused to make it so stable it will not react. One could relate this to a saturated fat. Another analogy might be the exposure of dry paper to sufficient heat to make it catch fire without any evident precipitating action. Heat itself can cause the chemical reaction in dry paper because the chemicals in that paper are easily available for oxidation at high temperatures. The difference between striking the match, and the self-igniting paper, is that the usually dormant paper *auto*-oxidizes; that is, it performs its chemical reaction spontaneously, the heat alone acting as a catalyst, or precipitating factor, to cause the ignition of the paper's chemicals with the oxygen in the air.

So it is with polyunsaturates. They are so unstable that the slightest trace of a catalyst can cause that particular fat to autooxidize and begin its chemical reaction in the body. Some easily available catalysts that will initiate the destructive process of polyunsaturate oxidation include the ozone or nitrous oxide that is always in smog; any form of radiant energy such as x-rays, cosmic rays in the air and even sunlight; the heating of polyunsaturates, as is necessary when they are used in cooking; and even certain trace metals such as iron, which is normally found in abundance in the body. Once the process starts, the polyunsaturate breaks down into what is known as free-radical compounds which then automatically combine with the oxygen in the body. These chemical compounds are then really toxic substances (sometimes called peroxides) and are known to damage and destroy body cells, the components within those cells and other body proteins such as the chromosomes.

The end-result of this chemical reaction in the body, which can be seen and measured under the microscope, is the ceroid, or aging pigment (sometimes referred to as a lipofuscin pigment, the "lipo" referring to its fat content.) And the ceroid pigment that results is really the dead body cell which can no longer function as it should. It does not seem inappropriate to say that anything that causes more ceroid bodies (clinkers) in tissues—faster than the body would ordinarily produce them—will also cause premature aging as well as diseases that accompany, or are the result of, premature aging. And it is known that the greater the amount of polyunsaturates in the body, the greater the amount of "clinkers" that occur. It has also been proven that the more polyunsaturates in the tissues, the more they are available for oxidation and eventual destruction of healthy active cells. Thinking back to the boy with the ruptured spleen, the excessive amounts of polyunsaturates eaten seemed to be the only cause of the fragility and eventual destruction of his spleen.

Even those who advocate an increased amount of polyunsaturates in the diet, such as Dr. Theodore Cooper, director of the National Heart and Lung Institute, admit polyunsaturates form peroxides and "are producers of free radicals which can produce local tissue damage."

That foods themselves can have severe side-effects in humans is certainly not new. Too much sugar can be "toxic" to a person with diabetes; too much salt can be quite dangerous to a person with high blood pressure; and even cheese, chocolate or pickled herring can cause a catastrophic chemical reaction in a patient taking a particular type of antidepressant drug called a monoamine oxidase inhibitor. It is not out-of-place, therefore, to look with great concern on any food that has already shown how dangerous it can be. To be sure, in the case of polyunsaturates, as with vitamins A and D, a small amount in the diet *is* necessary and they are only harmful when taken to excess.

But more and more people *are* taking polyunsaturates to excess. Studies have shown that millions of Americans are purposely altering their diets in order to eat as much of the polyunsaturated fats as possible—even to the extreme of swallowing tablespoonsful of oil directly from the bottle. These people are not even considering the amount of extra calories, and therefore extra weight they are adding with such a regime. And extra weight can be far more dangerous to a person's general health, as well as his heart, than cholesterol in the diet. With so much evidence of possible dangers, one wonders why Dr. Fredrick J. Stare of the Nutrition Department of Harvard has suggested in his newspaper column that one might well take three tablespoonsful of ordinary polyunsaturated cooking oils a day as a "medication" in order to keep one's cholesterol level down. He has repeatedly advocated a marked increase in polyunsaturates for everyone, along with a severe reduction in foods containing cholesterol.*

This type of blanket medical advice is given without consideration of individual differences or individual needs; without even examining the person being prescribed for (which is illegal in most states). As a result of such arbitrary and capricious recommendations, and as a result of the concerted efforts of advertisers to influence people to buy a food product to be used as a medicine —even without an established physical need or doctor's recommendation—a great number of people have deliberately altered their diets, feeling compelled to eat as much polyunsaturated oil as they can swallow without gagging.

* And yet the same Dr. Stare has publicly stated: "I don't know anyone who works in this field who has ever said that high cholesterol diets, or more correctly, diets that elevate the level of cholesterol in the blood, cause heart attacks." The contradiction in itself is cause for suspicion.

Dietary surveys have shown that at the very least two out of every five patients questioned concerning their diets admit to purposely substituting commercial products advertised to be "high in polyunsaturates" for such nutritionally valuable foods as meat, eggs and dairy foods. What is even more culpable though, is that in the same type of survey nine out of ten of those who have altered their daily food patterns also admit they did so without the advice or knowledge of their doctors. Most of those questioned said they changed their eating patterns as the result of advertising by industries that profit from their purchases, or as the result of publicity from the American Heart Association— which ultimately profits by a person's fear. Many physicians wonder why the Heart Association promotes the excessive use of polyunsaturates when even some of the research they have funded shows either the ineffectiveness, or harm of such a regime. Why have they suppressed these reports in favor of those promoting polyunsaturates?

The primary provocation to increase the amount of polyunsaturates in the diet seems to come from the advertising of those who sell such fats and oils for profit. As the U.S. Department of Agriculture figures reveal, these industries have been most successful in their commerical campaigns. The amount of polyunsaturates bought by the "average" person has increased almost three-fold over the past few decades, from about two percent of the diet in the early fifties to about six percent today. Those who have been "converted" to the polyunsaturate dogma, however, eat well over ten percent of their diets in these fats each day; some people quite intentionally eat more than twenty percent as a routine part of their diets.

Even though it is almost impossible to find a generalized population on this earth that "normally" eats more than ten percent polyunsaturates in their diet, the American Heart Association diet booklets will, if followed, lead one to eat, on the average, at least fifteen percent of one's food in polyunsaturated fat. And this without definitive proof that such a diet will prevent or cure heart disease, let alone a cautionary note about what happens chemically when these recommended fats are heated. Many physicians considered experts in the field of heart disease have warned that no one should eat more than 10 percent polyunsaturates in the diet. Yet, this fact is rarely brought to the public's attention.

What can happen when the polyunsaturate content of the diet is increased beyond the small amount (less than one percent) which the body needs? Although much of the research has been conducted on animals (animal experiments first showed the dangers of cyclamates, certain birth control pills and other drugs), unfortunately there has been a great deal of evidence in humans, too, to indicate that too much of the polyunsaturated fatty acids can be more dangerous than the conditions which these fats are supposed to prevent and treat. As a matter of fact, some doctors have quite pointedly shown that the use of polyunsaturates can cause more heart and artery disease than it is supposed to cure. But strangely these studies are never brought to the public's attention as are those that favor polyunsaturates.

Two of the most grievous findings that have been suggested by studies of the excessive use of polyunsaturates are premature aging and the shortening of the life span. Dr. Denham Harman, professor of medicine and biochemistry at the University of Nebraska College of Medicine, not only reports that the more unsaturated a fat is, the more it seems to *increase* the possibility of atherosclerosis, cancer and other disease; he also shows that the more polyunsaturates he feeds animals, the sooner they die. On translating his findings in animals to humans, Dr. Harman feels that the concentrated use of polyunsaturates can shorten man's life span by 15 years.

To find out if such an observation could be related to humans, a study of premature aging was made with the cooperation of the Research Foundation for Plastic Surgery in Los Angeles. Over a two-year period, more than one thousand patients were observed for any pathological evidence that they had grown old prematurely, as well as for the amount of skin growths that they had had removed. In order that knowledge of the patient's diet could be of no influence, the patient filled out a dietary survey which was withheld from the examining physician (a prominent Beverly Hills, California, plastic surgeon, Dr. Cadvan O. Griffiths, Jr.). This dietary survey undertook to discover whether the patient had changed his diet to stress polyunsaturates, to what extent, and for what reasons. The physical evaluation of the patient and the dietary survey were correlated at a later date by a third researcher.

Obviously many patients who come to a plastic surgeon are concerned about how old they look. But a great many patients also come for reconstructive surgery such as the cosmetic repair of tissues following accidents, burns, or the removal of ugly scars that often accompany a cancer operation. No matter what the reason for his or her visit, each consecutive patient who came to the plastic surgeon's office was evaluated by an objective scoring technique that could consistently indicate by repeatable standards the degree of damage to skin and underlying tissue that ordinarily accompanies aging.

The skin of the face was chosen for study of premature aging because of the ease of examining this area, as well as the accepted medical opinion that: "One of the most generally reliable and widespread clues we have to the age of individuals is the appearance of the skin during the aging process." In each patient, the degree and amount of wrinkles such as crow's feet, frown lines, etc.; skin turgor or firmness; color; elasticity or resilience; condition of the hair and many other factors which are significant signs to the practiced eye of the plastic surgeon, were measured and enumerated to attain a tentative total score. Then points were deducted from that total "aging" score if the patient had been exposed to a great deal of x-ray or sun; if one or both of the parents looked prematurely aged; if dentures were worn; or, if the patient suffered from any form of water retention (edema) such as swollen eyes in the morning or swollen ankles at night. Even excessive animation of the facial muscles was felt to contribute toward premature aging of the facial skin and was taken into account as a non-diet related cause.

Once all of the possible contributory factors in premature aging of the skin other than diet were noted, a final score was computed and this was compared with the patient's chronological age. The result was that of those who admitted to being on a diet high in polyunsaturates (more than 10 percent of the diet), at least 78 percent showed marked signs of premature aging of the skin of the face; some actually appearing more than 20 years older then they were. When this group was compared to an almost equal number of those who made no special effort to eat polyunsaturates, the difference was profound. Only 18 percent of the latter group were judged to have outward physical signs of premature aging. In other words, there were more than four times as many people who looked markedly older than they really were in the group that intentionally stressed large quantities of polyunsaturates in their diets.

To be sure, there can always be some question as to how old a person really looks, albeit no one is better qualified to make this sort of evaluation than a plastic surgeon. But there was a very dramatic coincidental finding of the study that seemed to more than confirm the matter of premature aging. For, just as the condition of the skin is considered a reliable clue to aging, so does the medical profession know that as skin becomes older there is an increase in skin growths that tend to become malignant (cancerous or precancerous). And when the same patients who were evaluated for premature aging were also asked if they had any skin growths removed since they had gone on a high polyunsaturate diet, 60 percent said they had had at least one, and sometimes more skin lesions removed surgically. In contrast, of those who had not altered their diets to stress polyunsaturates, only 8 percent had undergone skin surgery for growths. More than seven times as many people on an excessive polyunsaturate diet had had skin growths removed.

Other serendipitous, but none the less ominous, observations came out of the study. Some patients were found to be anemic; they complained of fatigue, and they looked quite pale. Two women felt they were short of breath and one man had had his surgery deferred because of anginal pains. As is the usual procedure, each patient with anemia was examined first to locate some sources of internal bleeding, the most common cause of anemia. In three patients none could be found. The dietary survey, however, did show that these people had altered their diets to eliminate all meat and eggs and increased their intake of polyunsaturates in the firm belief that they were protecting their hearts. A more detailed evaluation of the diet showed that all of these patients ate less than 5 mg. of iron each day (less than half that recommended as the very minimum daily requirement) by virtue of the fact that they avoided foods naturally rich in iron. In each of these cases, once the diet was restored to normal (balanced), the iron deficiency anemia disappeared and the symptoms that resulted from the anemia (including the anginal pains) also disappeared. The most common cause of folic acid (a vitamin) anemia in man comes about when people do not eat sufficient meat or related products.

Quite a number of patients in the study commented on the fact that they had swollen ankles at night and/or swelling of the face and eyes in the morning. The plastic surgeon evaluating the manifestations of aging strongly believes that water retention in any form is a widespread precipitating cause of aging skin. A careful evaluation of many of the edematous patients offered no other diagnostic finding than a low total serum protein when tested in the laboratory. While such a test could be indicative of certain disease conditions, it also reflects a diet unusually low in proteins.

Again in reviewing the diet history, it was found that where a good many patients had purposely increased the amount of polyunsaturated fats in their diets, they had also decreased the amount of proteins they ate each day. Two patients stated that they substituted several tablespoons of a polyunsaturated oil (as suggested in a medical diet-advice column) taken directly in place of meat, dairy products and eggs. When the polyunsaturates were reduced and a balanced diet restored, most of the patients who had recently developed water retention no longer complained of the same degree of swelling of the feet and face.

Another study that has been reported in the medical literature, but not publicized, concerns a group of patients who were told to substitute polyunsaturated fats for saturated fats wherever possible in their diets. After these patients had been on their diets for several months (they used the American Heart Association's booklet on fat-controlled meals as a guide) a few conclusions were possible. First, these test-people had raised their intake of polyunsaturates from an average of five to an average of 15 percent of their diets (15 percent was the mean reported by the study's dietician; many were eating a much greater amount). Second, they ate fewer proteins, but they did increase their amount of carbohydrates (sugars, starches, etc.). The more polyunsaturates the patients ate, the more polyunsaturates (in higher concentrations than normal) were found stored in their tissues. Furthermore, the results of the laboratory test for uric acid (usually associated with gout, but also known to reflect the destruction of protein in the body) were significantly increased in every patient whose diet included excessive polyunsaturates. Uric acid increases in the body following tissue damage and cell destruction. To have the serum uric acid rise (called hyperuricemia) in patients who were eating increased polyunsaturates is as yet unexplained, but an elevated serum uric acid is a definitive warning sign that something is wrong within the body.

The American Heart Association has made the statement that an elevated serum uric acid is a definitive heart disease risk factor, and in studies of patients with known coronary heart disease, more of these patients have elevated serum uric acid levels than they have elevated cholesterol levels. Therefore, if excessive polyunsaturates do cause one's serum uric acid level to rise, this, too, could be a definitive clinical indication that these particular fats might do more harm than good.

Some of the studies on animals given polyunsaturates (not necessarily in large amounts) have shown shortening of the life span, premature aging, and development of high blood pressure. When animals have been fed diets of lard they seem to have the lowest blood pressure. The more polyunsaturates that are fed, the higher the blood pressure seems to go. As somewhat of an aside, albeit still directly related to the problem, once a person has some evidence of heart disease it is not unusual for him to go on a high polyunsaturated diet because he has been influenced by all of the publicity on the subject. This, in itself, could be a potentiating factor in the frequency of the development of high blood pressure *after* the first indication of heart disease.

Another specific disease that has developed after animals have been given diets of polyunsaturates (and not necessarily diets that are abnormally high in this type of fat) is amyloidosis, a condition where gelatin-like material, usually protein-related, is deposited in various parts of the body. It is believed that amyloidosis may be a cause of senility, arthritis and other chronic conditions. Many animals develop cirrhosis of the liver almost identical to that caused by too much alcohol, after eating excessive polyunsaturates. And experiment after experiment has shown that feeding various polyunsaturates such as corn oil can cause more heart and artery disease than it is supposed to cure.

When the diet of cats contains excessive polyunsaturates, the cats develop steatitis—sometimes called yellow fat disease—

where the fatty layer just under the skin becomes agonizingly painful if touched, even ever so lightly. Cats on a balanced diet have never contracted this condition.

One fairly consistent observation in animals who are fed polyunsaturates compared to animals fed saturated fats, is that those who eat more of the polyunsaturates almost always develop diarrhea, lose hair, fail to grow, and far more often that would be expected, die within a matter of days or weeks. A proven effect of corn oil in the diet of animals shows that the more corn oil that is given the less the liver has the ability to detoxify certain drugs such as the barbiturates. And it is generally agreed by scientists everywhere that any increase in polyunsaturates in the diet requires an increase in the amount of vitamin E that must be taken into the body. Severe blood diseases have already been diagnosed in human infants as a consequence of a diet high in polyunsaturates along with a lack of sufficient vitamin E.

Some polyunsaturate advocates have urged, without scientific justification and without regard to the harm that may result, that: "The 'holy' value of milk should be deemphasized" and polyunsaturates substituted for milk from the time of birth. The Commission on Nutrition of the American Academy of Pediatrics has responded to such unwarrantable proposals that: "results of studies in which dietary cholesterol was limited in hopes of reducing the frequency of coronary heart disease are still far from convincing." Dr. Nathan J. Smith, a pediatrician at the University of Washington and an expert in infant nutrition, has said it is prudent "to resist the temptation to radically alter the intake of dietary fat in the first year of life. There is no assurance of beneficial effect from a low-fat infant diet in regard to the development of obesity or atherosclerosis." And there is always that doubt as to what might happen to the brain of a child during its growth stage when cholesterol is a necessity (see Chapter 3).

Many other observations of toxicity due to excessive ingestion of polyunsaturates, once observed only in animals, are now being observed in humans. Doctors are reporting liver damage in people who have altered their diets in order to eat more polyunsaturates. In another study on men, increased amounts of polyunsaturates caused "sludging" of the blood; that is, the red blood cells clotted together and did not flow as freely as necessary to carry oxygen to the body tissues, sometimes totally interrupting the blood flow. There are some who now attribute much of the lung damage in areas where smog is a regular atmospheric pollutant to an increased amount of polyunsaturates in lung tissue that are acted on by the main ingredients of the smog.

Of course, the most detrimental effect of ingesting excessive amounts of polyunsaturates is their association with cancer. It is known that the more polyunsaturates one eats the more polysaturated fatty acids appear in the body tissues. In a study from the Mayo Clinic, it was shown that patients who have breast cancer also have an increased amount of polyunsaturates in their breast tissue as well as in their blood plasma. While this study was of humans, another doctor at the University of Western Ontario recently told the American Heart Association that the more polyunsaturates he fed his animals, the more breast cancer they developed. This consequence was also noted by Dr. Denham Harnum of the Nebraska College of Medicine. Such observations are not new, however. More than 10 years ago, the possible mechanism of excessive polyunsaturates causing cancer was presented in a medical journal article that discussed how these fats can disrupt normal cell division and possibly promote the cancerous activity of cells.

When two physicians at the Veteran's Hospital in West Los Angeles experimented for eight years on two groups of men, giving one group four times as much polyunsaturated fatty acid as the second group, the end result was that those on the increased polyunsaturate diet had 60 percent more cancers than those who ate a regular balanced diet. Since this report was published in 1971, there have been four other studies throughout the world involved with the relationship of polyunsaturate intake to cancer. When the total number of patients involved in all of the studies were reviewed, those taking increased polyunsaturates had one-third more cancer than those eating a normal amount of different kinds of fats. A summary report of the five studies also stipulated "that the life-saving potential of serum cholesterol lowering diets is not proven."

In those countries where fish, which is high in polyunsaturates, is a staple of the average diet, there is a related increase in stomach cancer. Japan, for example, has the highest incidence of stomach cancer in the world. Next come people who live along the coast of Sweden and Finland where fish is one of the primary foods. As if to reinforce the relationship between polyunsaturates and cancer, there has been a recent study to show that where the diet is low in eggs, meat and dairy products, there is an unusually high incidence of esophageal cancer.

Along the same lines, Dr. Henry Eyring of the University of Utah (who is a National Medal of Science recipient) feels that anything that generates "free-radicals" as polyunsaturates do, also causes chromosome damage, which may well lead to cancer. Dr. Eyring says: "It might also be possible to gain several more years of good health by avoiding foods known to contain substances that can damage chromosomes."

Many more medical reports could be cited to show the relationship between excessive polyunsaturates and cancer as well as other degenerative conditions. But at this point, attention should be called to the additional danger of heating polyunsaturates. When a polyunsaturated fat or oil is heated, there is a chemical action that causes the polyunsaturate to act with the oxygen in the air and form a polymer or a new chemical compound that is usually the same chemical multiplied manyfold. Plastics are polymers. Varnish and shellac are polymers. In fact, it is the heating of polyunsaturated oil that produces varnish. That polyunsaturates form varnish in the body was demonstrated when animals that were fed such heated fats were found the next morning stuck to their cage floors by their varnish feces. Some of the animals suffered total intestinal obstruction from the polymerized polyunsaturates.

When animals were fed heated polyunsaturates and heated butter to note the effect on their health, the animals fed the heated corn oil had markedly lower growth rates, developed diarrhea and their fur became rough. All of the animals given heated corn oil developed tumors, and only one of the original 96 survived the 40 month experimental period. In contrast, none of the animals fed heated butter developed tumors and all survived.

When a polyunsaturate is heated it acquires a new, lower, iodine number. The iodine number is the way fats are determined to be saturated or unsaturated. The lower the number the more saturated the fat is supposed to be. Thus, cooking polyunsaturates lowers their iodine number and, therefore, they could be thought of as more saturated; another fact which seems to be ignored by those promoting cooking with polyunsaturates as a preventive or cure for heart disease.

Dr. David Kritchevsky, of the Wistar Institute in Pennsylvania, has demonstrated that when corn oil is heated for no more than 15 minutes and then fed to animals, it actually enhances rather than reduces atherosclerosis. Yet no one warns the public not to cook with these oils.

The longer a polyunsaturated fat or oil is heated, the more dangerous it becomes. Think of this the next time you visit a commercial establishment that deep-fries its foods. Almost all of these food suppliers re-use their cooking oil. They only add new oil to the vat to maintain the proper cooking level, as the old oil is withdrawn on the foods that have been cooked. In Germany, the re-use of cooking oil in a commercial establishment for more than three days resulted in the imprisonment and harsh fine of the restaurant owner.

In one experiment performed by Dr. Daniel Melnick and his colleagues at CPC, International (formerly known as Corn Products Company), the heating of corn oil raised the amount of a component (DNUA fraction) of that oil three times the amount that was present before the oil was heated. After his heated oil was fed to animals, the female animals had a 127 percent increase in breast cancer. In the same experiment, when a saturated fat was subjected to the same heat treatment and then fed to similar animals, the amount of breast cancer was not increased at all, and these animals lived much longer.

Dr. Roslyn Alfin-Slater, of the University of California at Los Angeles, showed that the feeding of heated polyunsaturates interfered with the reproductive performance of animals. And, Dr. A. L. Tappel of the University of California at Davis has demonstrated testicle damage in animals fed excessive polyunsaturates, due to the high concentration of polyunsaturates absorbed by these organs. Surprisingly, the amount of heated polyunsaturates that caused the damage rarely was more than 10 percent of the diet. In one particular study, when the amount was raised to 15 percent of the diet, all of the animals died within three weeks.

In a report delivered to the American Heart Association in November, 1970, (but never publicized to the public or the medical profession), Dr. Neil R. Artman of the Proctor & Gamble Company admitted that polyunsaturated fats can be made nutritionally undesirable by any conditions of heating and oxidation. Saturated fats, on the other hand, give no appreciable reaction to heat and air. The initial products following heating are peroxides, which are toxic. Dr. Artman stated that when polyunsaturates are heated in air (as in normal cooking): "linolenate is largely converted to polymers or varnish." He went on to say that "The most abusive conditions occur in deep fat frying in some restaurants, where the fat is kept hot for long periods often times for many hours without having food fried in it. . . ." He called such restaurant fat the worst fat that we are likely to be exposed to in our diets.

In addition to the dangers from heating polyunsaturated oils, another finding by the Food and Drug Administration, that was never made public, showed that in the commercial processing of polyunsaturated oils there was a tendency for the oil to hold any dangerous insecticides that may have been on the original vegetable from which the oil was extracted. In most instances chemicals similar to gasoline are used to extract the oil from the vegetables (corn, soy beans, etc.) and these petroleum products tend to hold onto the toxic insecticides that may be present before processing, thus contaminating the final product.

Another potential danger in commercially produced polyunsaturated margarines and oils is the addition of the chemicals BHT and BHA to the oils to give them a longer shelf life. Neither so-called "freshness preserver" has been effectively ruled out as a cause of cancer, and both have recently been shown to cause brain damage.

In spite of all the inferential evidence of harm to animals, as well as the harm now increasingly appearing in humans, very little is being done by those government agencies whose task it is to protect the public. When only one species of animal developed dangerous signs after taking a particular brand of birth control pill, the FDA warned all physicians to stop prescribing that pill and requested the pharmaceutical company to stop advertising and selling its product. The same warning came for various other food and drug products after they were shown to have dangerous effects on animals. But nothing has been brought to the public's attention about the potential dangers of polyunsaturates—especially when taken to excess.

Commercial interests, with little knowledge of clinical medicine and no evident concern for the individual harm they might be causing, have been and still are prescribing polyunsaturates as a therapeutic agent as if they were doctors prescribing a medicine. These corporations or health agencies never examine individuals, nor have they ever clinically proved the need for, or effectiveness of, this particular form of food they are recommending to be used as a drug. Even though this type of fat is, in reality, being recommended as a "medication" for disease, the normal government standards usually required to determine the *safety* of such a "prescription" have, strangely, not been considered. One wonders why the FDA and the FTC have overlooked the flagrant violations of laws by these industries.

CHAPTER *6*

THE GOVERNMENT VS. THE
CONSUMER IN THE MATTER OF
CHOLESTEROL

"MY MOTHER IS killing me—making me eat two eggs and bacon and toast with butter for breakfast." This was what an eighth grade boy said after taking a health course taught through a government sponsored health education program in a public school near Albany, New York. Children in other New York state schools and in Illinois, are regularly being told that their parent's proven ideas of good nutrition—valuable high protein meals at the start of the day—are more a deliberate means of hurting them rather than helping them. These newly-turned teenagers are being told that cholesterol is the cause of heart disease and that eating cholesterol, as well as saturated fats, is as fatal as cyanide or arsenic. They are also being taught that by substituting polyunsaturates in their diets they can prevent heart disease—something no one really knows and something that, after three decades of intricate study, has never been proven.

The government bureau that sponsors the deceptive teaching in New York is not alone. Many federal agencies have also turned their backs on such dissembling, ignoring the public's well-being that they allegedly exist to protect.

Dr. Charles C. Edwards, commissioner of the Food and Drug Administration, has stated that *if* his agency had the responsibility to protect the public from the false and misleading advertising of polyunsaturated products now appearing in contemporary magazines, newspapers and professional medical journals, he would regard those products as "misbranded" and would sieze them. The FDA regards as illegal the present type of advertising that pointedly makes, or simply alludes to, claims that polyunsaturates will lower cholesterol, and therefore will prevent or treat a heart attack. As a matter of fact, the FDA has publicly stated that such advertising has been illegal since 1959, but to date it has never taken any official action against any of the many flagrant violators.

Even though the FDA is specifically charged with protecting the consumer from fraudulent health claims, the agency takes refuge in the excuse that such advertising is the sole province of the Federal Trade Commission and therefore, the FDA has no responsibility, either moral or legal, to see to it that the consumer is not defrauded by unsubstantiated health claims for foods. It is up to the FTC, the FDA says, and then ignores the whole matter. But, says the FDA, should the *label* (as opposed to the advertisement) on a food carry any misleading or illegal statement, then it could act. However, even though many labels do, in fact, carry wording absolutely contrary to FDA regulations, the FDA still refuses to act. And the consumer is misled because the very regulatory agency established to protect him, refuses to carry out its *raison d'être.*

It is not that the FDA does absolutely nothing. It is simply that the FDA is selective, totally ignoring those violations it chooses to ignore. For example, it passes the buck to the FTC on polyunsaturate advertising, saying polyunsaturates are a food, but if they were a drug it would have jurisdiction. The fact that polyunsaturates are a food recommended to be used as a drug, the FDA chooses to ignore.

The FDA requires that any drug advertised to lower cholesterol must carry a notice to the effect that no one knows what the ultimate effects of such a drug are; that the drug could even be harmful. Furthermore, drugs to lower cholesterol must, according to FDA regulations, be accompanied by "An Important Note" (see page 18) that stipulates that no one knows if drug-induced cholesterol lowering will have any effect—good or bad—on heart disease. No such disclaimer, however, is required on the polyunsaturates sold for the identical purpose.

If a food is advertised in such a way that its use can be construed as a drug to prevent or cure heart disease (as in the case of polyunsaturates), existing law actually puts that food under FDA jurisdiction. But in the matter of polyunsaturates the FDA has relinquished its responsibility to the FTC.

Take a look at the law, published in 1959 that specifically indicts misleading food advertising:

Title 21, Code of Federal Regulations, section 3.41:

> *Status of articles offered to the general public for the control or reduction of blood cholesterol levels and for the prevention and treatment of heart and artery disease under the Federal Food, Drug, and Cosmetic Act.*
>
> (a) There is much public interest and speculation about the effect of various fatty foods on blood cholesterol and the relationship between blood cholesterol levels and diseases of the heart and arteries. The general public has come to associate the term "cholesterol" with these diseases. A number of common food fats and oils and some other forms of fatty substances are being offered to the general public as being of value in the control or reduction of blood cholesterol levels and for the prevention or treatment of diseases of the heart or arteries.
>
> (b) The role of cholesterol in heart and artery diseases has not been established. A causal relationship between blood cholesterol levels and these diseases has not been proved. The advisability of making extensive changes in the nature of the dietary fat intake of the people of this country has not been demonstrated.
>
> (c) It is therefore the opinion of the Food and Drug Administration that any claim, direct or implied, in the labelling of fats and oils or other fatty substances offered to the general public that they will prevent, mitigate, or cure diseases of the heart or arteries is false or misleading, and constitutes misbranding within the meaning of the Federal Food, Drug, and Cosmetic Act. (Sec.403 (a),52 Stat.1047:21 U.S.C.343(a)) [24 F.R. 9990, Dec. 10, 1959] Restated, and reenforced in the Federal Register June 15, 1971.

And as if this statement was not clear enough, in May, 1964, the commissioner of the Food and Drug Administration publicly reiterated that law, saying that the FDA had decided "to proceed against the health claims made for vegetable oil products [polyunsaturates] based on the results of a consumer survey on public understanding of current labeling of such products." The FDA commissioner went on to say that: "terms such as 'polyunsaturated,' 'unsaturated,' 'low in cholesterol,' and similar statements mislead many people to believe that these foods will reduce blood cholesterol and thus be effective in treating or preventing heart and artery disease." Even the claim that a product is "better for you because it is made from 100 percent golden corn oil" is to be considered misleading and, therefore, in violation of the law. But, to date, no regulatory action has been taken to stop the unproved claims even though in 1971 the Federal Register reported yet another restatement of this code.

Dr. Philip L. White, Secretary of the American Medical Association's Council on Foods and Nutrition, publicly stated in 1971: "We are all tired by now of the unending advertisements for oils and margarines that promise to clear our arteries in much the same way a drain cleaner works." Dr. White also rebuked the American Heart Association for its promotion of polyunsaturates because, he said, no one really has pinned down the relation of diet to heart disease. Yet the misleading advertising goes on and on, increasing with time. Moreover, the government agencies that are supposed to protect the consumer from false claims do absolutely nothing about the unscientific promises for polyunsaturated fats.

The American Medical Association has gone even further in its frank statements that appear in its official new book *AMA Drug Evaluation—1971*. (This book was published by the Council on Drugs, a completely separate division from the AMA Council on Foods and Nutrition.) It states that evidence of the effectiveness of linoleic acid (the active ingredient of polyunsaturates) is lacking insofar as reducing blood cholesterol levels is concerned, and, there is disagreement concerning the benefits to be gained by lowering the levels of blood cholesterol by any means. The Council on Drugs concludes that dietary treatment to lower cholesterol "is not acceptable to many patients and has not been completely successful."

A Public Statement, issued as a general news release by the American Medical Association on "Diet, Cholesterol, and Heart Disease," was headlined: *Latest Food Fad Is Wasted Effort*. The statement went on to say: "The anti-fat, anti-cholesterol fad is not just foolish and futile, however. It also carries some risk." In discussing the possible reduction of blood cholesterol by dietary regulation, the AMA warns the public: "Scientific reports linking cholesterol and heart attacks have touched off a new food fad among do-it-yourself Americans. But dieters who believe they can cut down their blood cholesterol without medical supervision are in for a rude awakening. It can't be done. It could even be dangerous to try." The AMA news release then went on to recommend milk, cheese, ice cream, meats, eggs and butter as a regular part of any well-balanced diet, even for "those on weight reduction regimens." As recently as August of 1972, Dr. Philip L. White reiterated the AMA's position.

While the AMA, through some of its departments decries the promotion of polyunsaturates as a health cure, AMA publications accept large sums of money for advertising that makes these unwarranted claims. Ironically, scientific articles in some of the same journals that carry the misleading advertisements say such claims have no merit or substantiation. Perhaps the best explanation for such a medical paradox, the advertising to doctors in medical journals of food and drugs that are ineffective or that might well result in harm to the patient, was expressed by Ernest B. Howard, M.D., the executive vice-president of the American Medical Association, when he said: "Advertising is the medical journal's principal source of revenue, and I hope it will continue for many years to come."

But the point here is not so much the contradictory action of medical journals in advertising drugs and food products that are not considered to have evidenced either safety or effectiveness, it is the lack of action by a governmental agency whose task it is to prosecute violations of the law. The matter of the misleading advertising to doctors of polyunsaturates that claim effectiveness in heart disease was brought to the attention of the FDA and FTC long before the 1972 annual AMA convention closed its doors. Despite the fact that the AMA meeting permitted commercial exhibits for polyunsaturates, which were in direct opposition to federal regulations, nothing was done to prevent their display. While many physicians ignore such unfounded claims, they do find it difficult to explain to their patients that they are acting in the patient's best interests. Patients often doubt their doctor's ability when he does not endorse or advise those margarines and oils which claim such miraculous medicinal properties. The definitive reports in the medical literature, such as the one that showed that patients who were forced to reduce their blood cholesterol after having a heart attack actually had a greater incidence of subsequent heart attacks than those who ate normally (as long as they did not overeat), are not read by patients, but the advertising of the polyunsaturate industries are.

The FDA's selectivity of enforcement is an enigma. If laws exist to protect the public from unfounded claims, ineffective products or dangerous substances, it is strange that the agency charged with enforcement of these laws selects only certain industries over which to exert their powers for public protection.

The Delaney Clause of the Federal Food and Drug Regulations says that you cannot add anything to a food that has been implicated (no matter how remotely) in causing cancer in animals. Cyclamates were removed from general use because it was suspected that they were a cause of cancer in rats. The FDA removed saccharin from the list of substances "generally regarded as safe" on the basis of a single study. That study was supported by the sugar industry and claimed that if humans drank 875 bottles of a saccharin "diet" soft drink per day, for several years, they might possibly develop a bladder tumor. Not necessarily a cancer, but a tumor; there is a difference. The study was based on feeding rats enough saccharin to constitute at least five percent of their diet. Although no rat did, in fact, develop a cancer, a few showed a tumor and this was sufficient for the FDA to create fear about a product that has been used by millions of people for many years.

If the Delaney Clause were to be equally enforced by the FDA, products containing polyunsaturates, too, should be removed from the "safe list." That animals develop cancers and then die if fed more than ten percent polyunsaturates (an amount *less* than that recommended by the American Heart Association) does not seem to influence the FDA at all. This observation of death from polyunsaturates is not just limited to a single study, as was the case when saccharin was banned; there have been hundreds of such studies in the medical and scientific literature.

As late as 1972 the FDA seized bottles of vitamin E and multivitamin tablets simply because they were labeled as a "dietary supplement." Such labeling was considered misleading, although the FDA also admitted that no danger was involved. At the same time, when certain polyunsaturate products have been advertised *and labeled* in direct contradiction to public law, the

FDA refuses to act, even if there is some possible danger involved.

There are some intriguing "coincidences" that must be pointed out in considering the obvious lack of regulatory agency action to protect, or at least to inform, the consumer about polyunsaturated fats and oils. In 1971, the general counsel for the FDA—the man in charge of prosecuting any violations of FDA regulations (including those of mislabeled polyunsaturated products)—left the FDA to become president of the Institute of Shortenings and Edible Oils (the primary public relations group for polyunsaturates). At the same time, the man who had been the legal representative of the edible oils companies suddenly became the general counsel of the FDA—the government's lawyer now in charge of regulating and disciplining the activities of his former clients. Congressman Benjamin S. Rosenthal of New York charged that the "musical chairs" switch "reeks of conflict of interests." Ralph Nader and Mrs. Ruth G. Desmond, president of the Federation of Homemakers, joined with Congressman Rosenthal in asking the Health, Education and Welfare Secretary to rescind the appointment, saying it was nothing more than "an Alphonse-and-Gaston mutual benefit act," but the switch in jobs went through without a hitch and still nothing has been done about illegal labeling and claims for polyunsaturated products—admittedly an FDA responsibility.

A year later, the deputy commissioner of the Food and Drug Administration resigned his post to become assistant to the chairman of CPC, International (Corn Products Company)—the company that stresses the polyunsaturates in its corn oil products. Incidentally, this type of executive shift from a government regulatory agency to the industry that agency is supposed to control, is not without precedent. The former head of the Institute of Shortening and Edible Oils (prior to 1971) was also an FDA commissioner before he, too, went into the executive ranks of the very industry he was supposed to police.

Government and politics seem more directly involved with the matter of polyunsaturates than one would imagine. A good example can be shown by following the 1972 presidential campaign of Senator George McGovern. In July, 1971, Senator McGovern announced he would hold hearings on the relation of diet to heart disease, and it was stated, at first, that he would only listen to the testimony of those who had already declared themselves on the side of the polyunsaturates. Those who scientifically questioned the idea that meat, eggs and dairy products might not be the cause of heart disease were not even asked to offer their opinions. Once certain facets of the dairy industry heard of the biased Senate hearings, they protested that both sides of the story should be given, and through the efforts of Senator Gaylord Nelson the hearings were indefinitely postponed. Many months later, when there was a chance for an impartial presentation of what was known and what was only suspected in the matter of certain fats and heart disease, Senator McGovern again postponed the hearings.

In 1972 the hearings were again scheduled, but once again Senator McGovern postponed the whole idea until after the Wisconsin presidential primary elections—Wisconsin being the nation's biggest producer of milk, butter and cheese. Then after Senator McGovern won the Wisconsin primary, those hearings that could adversely effect the dairy, egg and meat industries were shelved. The end result is that the polyunsaturate industry goes right on promoting their products as if they will prevent and treat heart disease, and no one stops them, or brings to the public's attention the lack of any scientific evidence for this drastic dietary change that might even be harmful.

But the government's involvement with polyunsaturates is not limited to allowing misleading promotion to continue despite its rules and regulations. The FDA, in an internal memo (not offered to the consumer), noted that dioxins (pesticides considered "one of the most toxic substances we ever tested" by an FDA scientist) were being found in margarines and in crude vegetable oils. The tiniest amount of these chemicals caused inordinately severe damage in animals. Monkeys developed heart, lung and reproductive organ damage and humans exposed to minute amounts of the chemical have complained of liver damage, abdominal pains and weight loss. Congressman Richard McCarthy of New York cites how the presence of these chemicals in foods is in violation of FDA regulations, but that no action has been taken about the lawbreaking.

One of the most flagrant examples of misleading advertising to be ignored by the government regulatory agencies was the

1972 Fleischmann margarine company advertisement that boldly proclaimed 3500 cardiologists at a medical meeting sat down to a meal especially featuring their margarine. Obviously the advertisement was to reinforce the public's belief that their particular margarine will help the heart, by implying that the 3500 cardiologists unanimously accepted this hypothesis. In actual fact, however, at no one time did more than 478 of these doctors (and their guests) ever sit down at a single meal to eat this particular margarine. Furthermore it was reported in a medical news journal that a good many physicians attending this meeting escaped to a local coffee shop for hamburgers and milkshakes. A news report quoted one cardiologist's comment: "They're taking all the fun out of the meetings." Yet, this misleading advertisement has been condoned by the FDA, the FTC, and even the AMA which carried the ad in its own publications.

In 1970, the Fleischmann margarine company ran an ad entitled "Should an 8-year-old worry about cholesterol," and indicated that if parents did, in fact, worry about cholesterol and would feed their children the advertised margarine they could lessen the risk of heart attacks. An immediate investigation as to the propriety of this ad was undertaken by the Federal Trade Commission. The general counsel of the FTC reported to a congressional committee that its investigation "to determine whether that ad and similar ads were in violation of any statutes" would be completed by the end of February, 1971. The "investigation" was never completed (at least as of the end of 1972) and, in fact, has been virtually abandoned. Meanwhile, margarine advertising that is even more gross in its claims to prevent heart disease is appearing with greater frequency than ever before.

Food manufacturers imply in their promotions that polyunsaturates are an ingredient of certain foods such as margarines, when, in truth, the word "polyunsaturate" is actually an adjective that describes certain kinds of fatty acids. For example, corn oil is not a polyunsaturated fat; rather, it is composed of many different fatty acids, only some of which are polyunsaturated. Furthermore, if corn oil is used to make a margarine, many of these polyunsaturated fats must be saturated in the process, which requires hardening, or hydrogenation, of the oil to give margarine a more solid consistency. Thus to put the amount of polyunsaturates on a label is obviously an oblique way of calling attention to a supposed food-drug effect on the heart and arteries.

An interesting aspect of the government's role in protecting the consumer from unsubstantiated commercial claims comes from a recent court decision that stresses the FDA's responsibility to require manufacturers to demonstrate *with substantial evidence* the *effectiveness* of drugs already on the market. The same standard should apply to the effectiveness of food products promoted for use as drugs. The court stated that testimonials, impressions and unsubstantiated subjective views by physicians do not constitute the kind of substantial evidence required by law. Only an adequate and well-controlled impartial clinical investigation could be considered acceptable to conform with existing regulations. Yet the FDA chooses to ignore the fact that there have been no adequate or well-controlled clinical investigations to *prove* that the eating of certain foods to lower one's cholesterol, or even the lowering of cholesterol itself, will have a beneficial effect on heart disease. Since the FDA forces a drug manufacturer to note this fact when he advertises his product to lower cholesterol, one wonders why the FDA looks the other way when a food manufacturer makes the identical claim in gross violation of the law.

That such claims are not rare can be illustrated further by the large chain of fish and poultry stores that advertised that their fresh fish and poultry "guard your heart with polyunsaturated fats." When this misleading advertising was brought to the attention of the appropriate regulatory agencies, the agencies again turned their backs.

The government's role in the matter of diet and heart disease is not limited to regulatory agencies. Hundreds of millions of tax dollars have been given away in the past 20 years to try and establish some link between dietary cholesterol, blood cholesterol and heart attacks. In all this time, no definitive scientific proof has ever been established. But, rather than admit the vulnerability of this hypothesis and begin looking in other directions for preventives and cures of heart disease, the Federal Government persists in spending more and more money in the same inefficacious areas.

On the one hand we pay taxes to support regulatory agencies to protect consumers—but these agencies refuse to enforce their own laws. On the other hand we pay taxes to support research that purports to prove theories which in the past 20 years have not lowered the death rate from heart disease. The taxpayer does not seem to be underwriting research so much as he is subsidizing certain segments of the food industry. Regulatory agencies that are supposed to protect the public seem more inclined to protect the industries they are charged with regulating. And the public is the scape-goat who is paying in many ways for the promotion of an unproved hypothesis, while the incidence of heart disease continues to rise.

CHAPTER 7

THE DAIRY INDUSTRY AND THE CHOLESTEROL CONTROVERSY

AS A DIRECT result of the cholesterol controversy, the sales of certain vegetable oil products have more than doubled. With the substitution of foods "high in polyunsaturates" for foods containing the supposedly villainous saturated fats, it was inevitable that some branches of the food industry would suffer.

In these days of aggressive public relations and advertising campaigns when even political candidates can be packaged and sold to the public like any other product, one cannot help but wonder at the passive acceptance by the dairy industry of the slurs against their products. And yet, for the last twenty years representatives of the dairy industry have literally sat by and allowed the aggressive oil industry practically to abolish dairy products from the American table. For example, the newest attack that has been mounted by the polyunsaturate pushers is to keep all babies from drinking whole milk; Even breast milk has been denounced as dangerous because of its fat content.

Not surprisingly, other authorities on the matter of heart disease have publicly commented on the "possum tactics of those assaulted industries." Dr. George Mann, a professor of medicine at Vanderbilt University and a career investigator of the National Heart and Lung Institute said that such maligned food purveyors as the dairy industry "do not appear to me to have responded as they might—or should" to the vegetable oil industry's "puny evidence backed up by dramatic Madison Avenue techniques" comprising a relentless campaign against the "best diet in human history."

Many of the so-called "scientific" studies that purport to prove the polyunsaturate point of view are, needless to say, sponsored either directly or indirectly by various segments of the edible oil industry. And yet, the representatives of the dairy industry seem content to sit in their ivory towers doing nothing. There has to be an answer to their seeming indifference, and there is.

But first, those other industries whose products are aligned with what the American Heart Association calls the "treacherous" dairy foods must be mentioned. Eggs are an excellent source of protein and other valuable nutrients that cannot easily be obtained elsewhere, and they are a marvelous aid to the dieter. They help him cut down on calories and still feel that he is not being starved. Yet, Dr. Fredrick J. Stare, a nutritionist who strongly champions some food industries while maligning others, has viciously attacked eggs and milk while advocating fish. In a folder written especially for the National Fisheries Institute, Dr. Stare erroneously claims that fish has less cholesterol than milk. Yet the dairy industry as a whole does nothing openly to refute this false and misleading information.

The meat industry, too, has not escaped attack. Increasing numbers of people do not eat meat at all because they feel that substituting fish and poultry for meat will save their hearts and add to their longevity. Meat has been condemned as a possible danger to the heart even though new evidence shows that many meat fats have no effect on blood cholesterol. And, in addition, there are adequate studies that show that beef and pork contain no more cholesterol than do fish fillets—which are so falsely touted as miraculously heart-saving.

Many restaurants and bakeries that once used only butter have markedly lowered the quality of their products, while increasing their profits, by switching to vegetable oils and margarines. These businesses use the excuse that "it is better for your heart," while leaving discriminating people with a diminishing number of places where they can go and be assured of the fine taste of unadulterated food. The trade newspaper "Supermarket News " recently did an in-depth report on "A company that has almost made a fetish of using only 93-score butter and other similar high quality ingredients in its frozen baked goods." That same company now uses vegetable shortenings in many of its products with the result that consumers have complained of the difference in taste and smell of their products.

But of all the different food industries that have been affected by the revolutionary changes in the American diet, the dairy industry stands in the forefront. Although all the facets of the dairy industry have a well organized network throughout the country that is supposed to represent them in an "educational" capacity, these representatives of the dairy industry seem to care very little about the denigration of dairy products. Worst of all, these spokesmen for the dairy industry seem to do nothing to contradict the misleading propaganda that serves only to destroy the public's confidence in milk and dairy products. Why?

The dairy industry's position on the matter of cholesterol and heart disease may best be summed up by a 1970 letter sent to all dairy product distributors by the Dairy Council of California in response to requests for information on cholesterol. It pointedly said: "Dairy Council is not anxious to light any fires under this controversial subject."

Even with a great deal of scientific evidence to refute some of the statements made about the dangers of dairy products, the dairy industry is not anxious "to light any fires." This is an extremely paradoxical attitude to take in the light of the fact that dairy foods, in general, contain far less cholesterol than do many of the foods being pushed as dairy food substitutes. For example, an ounce of whole milk contains about 3 milligrams of cholesterol; equivalent amounts of poultry contain five times as much, fish fillets contain six times as much and veal contains eight times as much, even though poultry, fish and veal are promoted for use in "low cholesterol" diets. And, there are some margarines being used in so-called heart protection diets that contain 10 times as much cholesterol as whole milk, three times as much as ice cream and the same amount as butter. Many dairy foods, then actually contain less fat and cholesterol than do the "special" foods being recommended as dairy substitutes supposedly to prevent and cure heart disease, yet the dairy industry does nothing to correct this misinformation.

Could this be because many dairy distributors also distribute polyunsaturate products at an even greater profit? Many dairy companies do market dairy substitute foods so that no matter which direction the public interest takes, the distributor will be sure to come out ahead. Only the dairy farmer, or producer, seems to bear the brunt of this profitable conflict of interests. But, for some reason, even the dairyman back on the farm does not seem to protest too much or too loudly. Could this be because the federal government buys all of the butter the dairyman cannot sell on the open market at a price far higher than what he could make by competing on the open market?

For many years the United States government has been paying farmers from 68 to 70 cents for each pound of "surplus" butter. Then the government sells that butter to other countries, such as Great Britain, for only 50 cents a pound, with the American taxpayer making up the difference in price. In other words, Americans actually pay 20 cents a pound so that other countries can have as much butter as they desire while Americans eat the "cheaper spread." The United States government seems to have no health misgivings about how much butter its foreign friends eat; it sold Britain 12 million pounds in one month. If, however, the government cannot sell the surplus butter at 50 cents a pound, the butter is simply discarded when it turns rancid, with the taxpayer footing the entire 70 cents per pound cost of this dairy subsidy.

Butter is not the only dairy product that the federal government buys as surplus to aid and abet the dairy industry. In 1971 the Department of Agriculture removed 7.3 billion pounds (more than three and a half billion quarts) of milk from the competitive market. Taxpayers paid for this milk, over and above what they bought for their own use.

The representatives of the dairy industry have united into an unusually powerful organization. Look what they were able to do to Senator George McGovern when he wanted to hold hearings on the hypothetical relation of diet (primarily dairy foods) to heart disease. In a CBS-TV news program (July 12, 1971), commentator Daniel Schorr reported that "The Dairy Industry is fighting for its life against the growing American worry about cholesterol. People are using about half as much whole milk and butter as they used to." (No mention was made of the fact that although there has been such a marked decrease in these foods, the heart disease rate has skyrocketed.) Mr. Schorr went

on to say that "there were some palpitations among dairy producers when they learned that Senator George McGovern's Nutrition Committee planned to hold a series of sessions on diet and
public health possibly leading to recommendations for a change
in the American diet." Suddenly, just prior to the Wisconsin
elections, the hearings were cancelled, and Mr. Schorr concluded:
"In this case the potential for pressure is obvious since the Wisconsin primary is crucial to Senator McGovern's presidential as-
pirations."

If the dairy industry is powerful enough to stop a Congressional hearing—a strictly negative act—why then has it not taken
a positive stand and attempted to educate the public on what is,
and what is not, known about dairy foods and heart disease?
Their actions would almost seem to indicate that they want to
suppress all relevant knowledge in this area. Are they afraid that
if something happens to change the status quo, they may lose
millions of dollars in subsidies?

Dr. Jean Mayer of Harvard has also cited the dairy industry
for exerting "formidable pressure" on congressmen to cancel
committee hearings. But, he also says that the dairy industry's
fears that milk products would be declared a major culprit are
unfounded. Yet, while in the middle of this controversy, the dairy
industry does virtually nothing to educate the public about the
truth of dairy food nutrients insofar as heart disease is concerned.
Hence, the polyunsaturate propaganda continues unimpaired.

Perhaps the dairy industry really is not worrying at all. For
as the magazine *The Washington Monthly* (May, 1971) puts it:
"The dairy lobby buys the cream of the congress." It is the dairy
lobby that has assured the dairy farmer that by law, whenever the
market price of manufacturing milk (that used for butter, cheese,
etc.) falls below the "support" price (that the taxpayer must, by
law, subsidize); the dairy farmer is guaranteed a place to sell his
product without competition at a guaranteed profit. As a result
of such government supports, the dairy farmer's gross income
reached a record high amount in 1971. Obviously the supposed
fear of milk products as allegedly related to heart disease makes
no difference to the dairy industry as long as tax money is available to keep profits up, whether the products are sold in the
marketplace or not.

The power of the dairy lobby was made evident when, in

1971, the Secretary of Agriculture publicly declared that there would be *no* increase in price supports to dairy farmers. Then, thirteen days later, the same secretary changed his mind and raised the guaranteed payment of taxpayer's money to dairy farmers by six percent. One important event occurred during those thirteen days, when at first there was a determination not to allow a rise in dairy subsidy payments and then there was a complete reversal of policy to increase the federal price support level for milk. Hundreds of thousands of dollars in campaign contributions were made to various Republican committees by the dairy industry. In return the dairy industry benefited by $700 million through a simple one cent per quart subsidy increase. The link between the two events was such that Ralph Nader, the consumer advocate, filed suit against the government for "improperly and unlawfully" increasing the amount of tax dollars to be paid to dairy farmers for products that they could not, or would not, sell on the open market.

And, in spite of Nader's contention that the 1971 price subsidy increase was a payoff for political contributions to Nixon, the dairy industry is, in 1972, asking for another, even greater increase in price supports for milk. Obviously the less milk and the fewer milk products that are sold on the open market, the more the dairy farmer makes through price subsidies —without any need to worry about the public's using less milk. Why should the dairy industry aggressively combat misleading advertising and publicity against its products when the government more than makes up for the public's lack of dairy product consumption?

In order for dairy products to compete on the open market the dairy industry would have to offer public refutations to the unscientific accusations made against their products. But why should they bother to compete when the taxpayer supports their evident apathy? The tax money spent to support the dairy industry's unwillingness to support itself is far, far greater than all the money now being spent on research to find a real cure for heart disease.

In 1970 it was reported that the dairy industry donated more than a million dollars to various political campaigns. In return, the industry received more than $300 million the following year from the government—just about the same amount as the Lockheed C-5A overrun cost the government and which a dairy country senator thought a scandal to taxpayers. In the first few months of 1972, dairymen contributed more than half a million dollars for political purposes. Mr. W. R. Griffiths, chairman of the American Milk [industry] Government Relations Committee told Frank Wright, who was writing a series of articles on the dairy lobby for the Minneapolis Tribune: "You've been around long enough to know you don't get nothing you don't pay for."

William A. Powell, president of Mid-American Dairymen wrote: "The facts of life are that the economic welfare of dairymen does depend a great deal on political action. If dairymen are to receive their fair share of the government financial pie that we all pay for, we must have friends in government."

Anyone who has read any of the booklets distributed by manufacturers of polyunsaturate products, or those who have simply seen the misleading advertising put out by the same companies, must wonder why the dairy industry allows itself to be attacked so vehemently and not refute—especially since it can—the charges against its products. The answer seems to lie in the fact that the dairy industry stands to profit no matter which way the consumer goes. And this alone seems sufficient reason not to compete on the open market. As long as government subsidizes an industry or group, there really is no reason to be part of the traditional competitive system. Profit is the name of the game and it does not seem to matter—even to the traditionally conservative farmer—how that profit is made, so long as it is made.

The American Medical Association has publicly stated that, in the matter of feminine hygiene sprays (which it says are no more effective than soap and water): "smart advertising has built a multi-million dollar industry on the public's exaggerated *fears* of body odors." The edible oil industry has done the same thing in regard to the public's fear of heart disease, at the same time condemning dairy products as the cause of such illness. The dairy industry has done nothing to alleviate the public's fear, and evidently will not do anything as long as the profits continue almost directly as a result of that fear campaign, with the taxpayer underwriting those profits.

Obviously the dairy industry could put sufficient pressure on such regulatory agencies as the Food and Drug Administration and the Federal Trade Commission for allowing misleading advertising—especially such advertising that implicitly condemns dairy products as the cause of heart disease. If they have sufficient political punch to obtain repeated subsidy increases, and to muzzle a United States senator, they must have the political power to insist on honest advertising. But the dairy industry does not really do anything to demand proof for the claims against its products. Rather, as an industry, it will make a few squeaky noises within its own organization at certain times as if it were upset, yet still do nothing to alter the public's opinion about the unscientific claims concerning diet and heart disease. One should, therefore, not only question the misleading promotion for polyunsaturates; one should also question the failure of the dairy industry to stop such misleading promotion. And, it seems the only way something will be done is to stop paying greater profits in tax money to dairy farmers so that they will have to compete on the open market.

PART **III**

WHAT ARE THE ANSWERS?

IF YOU WISH to liberate yourself from the panic over cholesterol, there are many alternatives. While the single most important approach to alleviating almost any disease is the reduction of stress, there are other, basic ways to help yourself avoid heart disease. A proper, well-balanced diet that goes hand in hand with physical fitness is a practical, sound beginning toward good health—especially the health of your heart. Better still is the elimination of constant worry about your heart, plus the restoration of relaxation and pleasure to your mealtimes. Enjoy food rather than fear it.

CHAPTER 8

DIET AND PHYSICAL FITNESS—YOU
NEED BOTH

THE AMERICAN HEART Association has recently made a policy statement that: "It is not proven that dietary modification can prevent arteriosclerotic heart disease in man." At the same time, the association is spending publicly donated money to push dietary as a heart disease preventive. This policy statement came after many years of study by many experts in the field of cardiology. Yet, the American Heart Association continues to print millions of booklets and diet sheets, continues to sponsor radio programs and motion pictures, and continues to advertise to both the medical profession and the public that heart disease can be prevented by substituting polyunsaturates for saturated fats in the diet.

At this point, it seems appropriate to mention some of the recent research regarding saturated fats. That these fats have become known as "fatal fats," is an example of the misleading propaganda that now prevails. One is told that meat fats are bad. Yet, even some of those who make this claim admit that the main saturated fatty acid in meat fat, stearic acid, really does not elevate blood cholesterol after all. Some researchers have even shown that stearic acid actually lowers blood cholesterol, and even lowers blood pressure. Yet, the American Heart Association and the manufacturers of polyunsaturates continue to indoctrinate the public that saturated fats are bad and that polyunsaturated oils are not only good; they are life-saving. They do not publicize the experiments that showed that atherosclerosis occurred with diets containing corn oil and no saturated fats. They do not tell of the people who eat far more saturated fats than Americans do and yet are essentially free from heart disease, even in old age.

Another subject the advocates of polyunsaturates rarely talk about is the fact that the more polyunsaturates one eats, the more vitamin E one requires in the diet. *The Medical Letter,* a non-profit, drug information sheet sent to doctor-subscribers, and considered a very cautious medical publication, admitted that the amount of vitamin E one ingests *must* be increased if there is any attempt to increase the polyunsaturates in the diet. Commercially prepared polyunsaturated oils tend to lose much, and sometimes all, of their natural vitamin E; even the preservatives added to retain that vitamin E may be more harmful than helpful.

It has been repeatedly shown that a diet high in polyunsaturates, which causes a depletion of vitamin E in the body, also causes abnormal blood conditions. The excessive polyunsaturates, without sufficient vitamin E, destroy red blood cells. Vitamin E, which acts as an antioxident, seems to offer some protection when given in adequate amounts. At Tulane University, a diet high in polyunsaturates that caused a depletion of vitamin E in the body, also was associated with liver disease. And, recent research at Duke University shows that vitamin E does help prevent the formation of toxic peroxides from polyunsaturates, especially in the presence of smog.

There have been many other studies to show how Vitamin E seems to protect against the damage caused by excessive polyunsaturates, but whether vitamin E will actually prevent premature aging or skin growths has yet to be proved.

There has been a great deal of medical research into the matter of whether being overweight really is a health hazard. A few academic doctors whose work is primarily limited to teaching, and who do not regularly see patients, have said that being overweight, in itself, is no health hazard. Yet, mortality statistics show, and most practicing physicians still feel, that obesity (or the strain of carrying around excessive pounds just as if one carried around a load of heavy stones) could be dangerous to one's health. In addition to the significant statistical association between high blood pressure and being overweight, it has been shown repeatedly that a loss in weight can lower one's blood pressure without the use of medicine.

This does not mean that *all* high blood pressure comes from being overweight, or that a weight loss alone is an absolute cure for hypertension; it does mean, however, that a known risk of heart disease might be reduced when one's weight is within "normal" limits. To be sure, there are many markedly overweight people without any illness whatsoever, but, in general, there is a clinical relationship between obesity and many diseases—especially heart trouble associated with high blood pressure. And yet, when studies are made to try and correlate the blood cholesterol test with high blood pressure and being overweight, no scientific relationship can be found. Being overweight will not necessarily cause high blood cholesterol levels, nor will high blood pressure.

Despite the fact that so-called cholesterol-lowering diets (diets high in polyunsaturated fats and low in animal fats, requiring the restriction of dairy products, eggs, fatty meats and shellfish, and the substitution of vegetable oils and soft "special" margarines for butter and other fats) are still being recommended, they just do not prevent heart attacks. Another American Heart Association recommendation seems totally oblivious to the statistical dangers of obesity, in its obvious preoccupation with pushing polyunsaturated oils. They suggest that 4 tablespoons of polyunsaturated oil (corn, cottonseed, soybean, sunflower seed oil) be taken every day, and this oil will supposedly counteract all of the so-called "bad" (saturated) fats that are "wrongly" eaten. The association advises that the oil be taken directly, or in salad dressings, mayonnaise, or cooked in foods. But, no matter how it is consumed, the oil constitutes 500 calories that you are exhorted to add to your diet every day. The American Heart Association says polyunsaturates should lower blood cholesterol, but they do not tell you that you have to have a ratio of more than twice as much polyunsaturates as saturates *simultaneously* to achieve even a temporary effect. More important, when excessive polyunsaturate diets are used for prolonged periods of time (more than six months) blood cholesterol has a tendency to start back up to its original level, no matter how strict one is about the types of fat one eats.

One major fact must be made clear. Whenever the diet is deliberately altered—no matter how severely, or peculiarly—the typical initial lowering of blood cholesterol is only about 10 to 15 percent—still less than an amount considered to be the normal "error" factor when performing a cholesterol test. In other words, there is really no *significant* lowering of one's blood cholesterol through the use of polyunsaturates, *per se;* there may, however, be an incidental secondary effect. The deleterious effect that such oils will have on sensitive taste buds by distorting the expected flavor and smell of foods causes the person with an educated palate to lose all pleasure in eating. Thus, due to a secondary loss of appetite a person will eat less, lose weight, and his cholesterol level might fall momentarily.

Eating should be a pleasure. It should be a time of replenishing the spirit as well as the body. If suddenly, every time you sit down to a meal its impaired flavor takes some enjoyment out of the meal; if each meal becomes a medical event focused on heart disease and its possible prevention, the heart-dieter is in danger of becoming a heart-neurotic.

According to a recent nutritional study, restaurant eating is on the increase. Americans now eat about one-third of their meals out, and by 1980 are expected to eat about half of their meals away from home. When one eats in a restaurant, the percentage of calories consumed in fat soars to 72 percent, as compared to 40 percent in the average diet. It is also difficult to remain on a diet when one is a guest in someone's home. The host or hostess too often becomes offended when the guest repeatedly refuses food. No wonder, then, that a recognizable symptom of the polyunsaturate dieter is his compulsion to eat out frequently. One patient while dining at a restaurant with his wife asked her why she could not get the kind of good French bread they serve in most restaurants. After trying innumerable brands and bakeries, the wife finally discovered that no matter what brand of French bread she served, it received praise when she served it with sweet butter instead of margarine. It is a small matter, but just one of the many joys that are lost unnecessarily on a polyunsaturate regime.

People who are heart-conscious at every meal may be doing themselves more harm than any diet could possibly help. Stress, no matter what the cause, is a known risk factor in heart disease.

Therefore, the stress of being denied the simple pleasure of enjoying one's food, or of being forced to think that the things you would enjoy will kill you, could be creating a greater heart-risk factor than any food.

Of course, contrasted to those made miserable by a rigid medical regime are those whose psychologic make-up enjoys martyrdom. They would feel unhappy if they were not denying themselves with the hope of saving their hearts. Abstemiousness allows them to feel sanctimonious every time they sit down to eat or give up some activity they formerly enjoyed. While these people revel in any diet because of the attention it directs toward them, most others are plagued by anxiety over the discipline and denial required in a rigid diet.

There are some people who just cannot give up ice cream. It is foolish, then, to demand that they do. Ice cream, taken in small quantities, will probably be less harmful than the compensatory nourishment that the dieter usually seeks. For, compensation seems to run concurrent with steady dieting. Just as the heavy smoker takes a drink every time he "needs" a cigarette, as a method of giving up smoking, so do most dieters search for substitute satisfactions. Studies have demonstrated that those dieters who give up fats often compensate with carbohydrates, defeating their supposed purpose. Dietary sugar causes blood fats to increase—in many instances far more than fatty foods—so those people who substitute simple carbohydrates and sugar for the missing fats in their diets end up right back where they started, except for the added factor of anxiety caused by the heart-conscious change in diet.

If we accept that weight control is a more effective form of preventive medicine than substitution of one kind of fat for another, we must look for the most effective and comfortable means to reduce total body weight.

Euripides called: "Moderation, the noblest gift of Heaven." Moderation in diet, the avoidance of all extremes, is still the best rule to follow. The people who eat a little bit of everything are not apt to be missing necessary nutrients; they will add to their pleasure in eating, and will probably be able to maintain a healthy, normal weight, without anxiety—at least over eating.

The most successful diet is the one that includes all kinds of foods but simply reduces the quantity of food usually eaten.

Drugs or bizarre crash diets may reduce weight dramatically, but such weight loss is usually only temporary and followed by rebound overeating. One-thousand-calorie-a-day diets, for instance, are so difficult to tolerate and so boring for any length of time that they are seldom followed long enough to maintain any weight loss. What is really needed to control obesity is a lifelong commitment to your own best interests. Motivated by a desire to look and feel your best, over the years, you can establish patterns of eating that will insure healthy weight maintenance.

Calories are units of energy; if you take in more food energy than you expend, you are going to gain weight. If you put out more energy than you take in, you will lose. For each 3500 calories you forego, you will lose one pound. If, for example, you should require 3000 calories a day to maintain your present weight, then on a 2000 calorie-a-day diet you will lose about two pounds a week. If you expend energy actively playing tennis an hour a day, you can afford to have a few more calories than you would if you remained sedentary.

In order to get all of the nutrients the body needs, food should be chosen from the following four groups *every day.*

MILK OR DAIRY GROUP
(supplies necessary proteins, amino acids, calcium and vitamins)

Children should have 3-4 cups of milk a day or their equivalent (can be whole milk, skim milk, evaporated milk or buttermilk).

Adults should have 2 cups of milk or their equivalent. (Skim milk, of course is better for all those who have to budget their calories).

As substitutes for milk, the following may be used:

½ cup ice cream = ¼ cup milk

1½ cups cottage cheese = 1 cup milk

1 inch cube cheddar cheese = ½ cup milk

MEAT GROUP
(supplies essential proteins, amino acids, iron and vitamins)
(one serving is considered by most dieticians to be 3½ oz.)

beef   chicken

                    Lamb   turkey
                    veal   liver (and other organ meats
                           are low in calories)
                    pork
As substitutes or equivalents the following may be used:
                    fish
                    eggs
                    cooked dry beans, peas or lentils
                    peanut butter (4 tablespoons)
                    nuts

A good diet should include two or more servings from this group every day.

VEGETABLE AND/OR FRUIT GROUP

dark green or deep yellow vegetables (string beans, peas, carrots, squash)
citrus fruit or juice, or tomato
potatos and other vegetables and fruit (corn, onions, apples, bananas, etc.)
(4 or more servings of approximately ½ cup each should be included every day in the diet).

BREAD AND CEREAL GROUP

bread or rolls (whole grain or enriched)
rice (enriched)
noodles (enriched)
spaghetti (enriched)
macaroni (enriched)
cereals (whole grain or enriched)
(One serving is equal to 1 slice of bread, ½ cup cooked cereal, rice, noodles, spaghetti, macaroni, or one ounce of ready-to-eat cereal.)

There are many ways to get weight down and to keep weight within the normal range without sacrificing either pleasure or necessary nutrients. The important factor is for the individual to find a diet he can stick to. Mass diets do not take into consideration individual, cultural or ethnic backgrounds or needs. For these reasons, the individual has to find a weight maintaining diet that best suits him, his background and his needs. Only then will he be able to stay on a diet that keeps him at a healthy weight.

According to the World Health Organization: "When a family emigrates, it will first change its habits of lodging, then clothing, then language. The last link with the old style of life remains the food it eats, the way food is prepared and even its psychological role . . .; this food link sometimes continues for generations in the new home." Just as Americans are a homogenous society made up of a blending of diverse elements, so has the American diet become an amalgamation of diverse tastes. All of us may include spaghetti, tacos, and Chinese food in our diets, but there are generally food links that linger from our family backgrounds. These tastes, these likes and dislikes are all too often ignored when we are handed a diet sheet to follow.

Beyond diet, prudent exercise is another aid in keeping weight within the range of normal. Exercise does far more than simple use of calories. When properly performed, it markedly increases one's health by increasing physical fitness: not the physical fitness demanded by schools, where how far you can jump or throw a ball seems to be more a mark of the school's prestige than a real interest in the student's health; but your own fitness, which improves circulation, keeps the blood vessels wide open, allows the body to use oxygen more effectively, keeps up the tone in the muscles and skin, and in general, keeps the human body running in top form.

What may be most surprising is how little "exercise" is really necessary to achieve physical fitness. For the average person, in reasonably good condition, 20 minutes per day is sufficient. This can easily be achieved by a brisk one mile walk each day. A few steps here and there will not suffice, the one mile daily walk should be taken at one time. The idea is to improve circulation and temporarily increase the body's use of oxygen over and above its routine requirements. In this way the body will not react adversely to any sudden increased metabolic demand. While the walking, in itself, will only use up about 250 calories, it is the physical fitness it creates that is important.

Strenuous exercise is not necessary to achieve physical

fitness. The strain of jogging, running, or other prolonged extreme physical exertion is not advisable without first having a stress electrocardiograph—especially if one is over 35, or has not been physically active for a long period of time. This test can indicate the response of the heart to all degrees of physical activity and will offer adequate warning to prevent any damage from physical stress. Physical fitness is not derived from the amount one strains at physical activities, but rather how regularly one utilizes as many body systems as possible.

If you eat the same amount of food and perform the same amount of exercise in middle age as you did when you were younger, you will still gain weight. For, as the body becomes older, the basal metabolic rate declines, and in order to compensate for this normal decline, one must eat less each day (at least 200 calories less), or exercise more (to burn up at least 200 calories more). Thus a one mile walk each day, without increasing the amount of food you eat, can compensate for the declining metabolic rate in aging.

In spite of the fact that the Masai of Africa eat far more saturated fats and cholesterol containing foods than Americans, they have a virtual absence of heart disease, even in old age. On the average, Masai (even those over 50 years of age) walk at least five miles a day. They do not exercise strenuously; much of their walking is in the tending of their herds or attending meetings. They do, however, walk regularly; and, measuring their physical fitness scientifically, they surpass the physical fitness of our top athletes.

On the average, a 150 pound sedentary person (not on a diet) eats from 2,000 to 3,000 calories per day. At the same time he uses up approximately 2,500 calories. Thus, it is easy to see how a person's weight can fluctuate depending on the balance between dietary intake and exercise. A very active worker or full-time athlete may eat, and use up, 6,000 calories a day. It is easy to obtain a book that indicates the calorie content of foods, and it is good preventive medicine to become aware of how many calories you eat. But to use up those same calories is a lot more difficult than most people imagine.

If you run steadily for an hour at a rate of 10 miles per hour (which can be quite a strain), you will use up close to 900 calories. A game of golf, assuming you actually walk over the course and do not use a golf-cart, approximates walking without playing golf. An hour of playing tennis, however, will only use up about 150 calories more than walking. And even if you swim for a whole mile in a half-hour's time, you will only burn up 50 calories more than if you walked for an hour; but, should you walk vigorously, the loss of calories is identical with the loss in swimming. Surprisingly, you can burn up more calories by gardening or doing housework for an hour than you can through athletic activities.

Another form of "exercise" is sex. Many men and women fear that sexual activities will cause a strain on the heart. Research at Western Reserve University has shown that there is little or no strain on one's heart while having sex. The heart does not beat that much faster that there is cause for worry; and, for the few seconds that it does, it does not exceed the exertion of a short brisk walk. The stress or anxiety produced by worrying about the potential dangers of sex are far more dangerous than sex itself. The anxiety that occurs over extramarital sex, however, where an illicit rendezvous or the fear of inability to perform adequately for someone who "does not understand you," brings on a much faster heart rate as well as an increase in blood pressure.

The best way to lose weight is diet *plus* exercise. However, if the cholesterol controversy still gnaws at you, if you are still afraid not to lower your blood cholesterol level regardless of the absence of any proof that by doing so you will help your heart, diet *plus* exercise could lower your blood cholesterol far more effectively than any change in fats. If you are not overweight and have no need to diet, achieving physical fitness alone will markedly lower your cholesterol. You will also firm up your skin and the rest of your body. As you lose weight, regardless of what kind of fat you eat, your blood cholesterol level will also decrease. This has been reported in medical studies when there was no attempt to change from saturated fats to polyunsaturated fats.

What you eat is important, but whether you enjoy eating can be even more important. The same goes for exercise to achieve physical fitness. This too, should not be a burden or a bore, but something that offers pleasure. More than anything else, try to eat a balanced diet—a little of everything, with no extremes at either end of the saturated-polyunsaturated scale. Moderation is the key to good health in diet and physical fitness.

DID YOU KNOW . . .

¶ Measure for measure, fish has more cholesterol than ice cream?

¶ Measure for measure, veal has more cholesterol than fish, milk, or ice cream?

¶ Most margarines have almost as much saturated fat in them as butter?

¶ Skim milk contains cholesterol?

¶ The primary fatty acid that makes up the fat of beef (stearic acid) has no effect in raising, but may actually lower, serum cholesterol?

¶ Whipped butter has about 50 percent fewer calories than regular butter?

¶ Wine loses calories while cooking (it also loses alcohol, but not its nutrients)?

¶ Eggs are a wonderful diet food; they supply a large amount of protein and other nutrients not easily available elsewhere and are very low in calories?

¶ Diets low in protein may cause water retention, body swelling, and anemia?

¶ Fats delay the onset of hunger?

¶ Polyunsaturated oils have 25 percent more calories than butter?

¶ Heating polyunsaturated cooking oil causes it to polymerize (become saturated) and eventually become varnish?

¶ Fats carry fat-soluble vitamins; without fats your body cannot effectively absorb or use vitamins A, D, E, and K?

¶ Sugar alone can stimulate the production of fat in the body—apart from the calories it contributes to the diet?

¶ Olive oil is a monounsaturated fat; it has no effect on blood cholesterol levels?

CHAPTER 9

DRUGS, CHOLESTEROL, AND HEART DISEASE

THE WORD "DIET" usually has terrible connotations for those who need it most. If they did not love food, they would not need to diet. Because the dietary regulation of cholesterol, through a high polyunsaturate diet, is not universally successful, and potentially dangerous and because cutting down on calories can be so unpleasant to a lover of good food, people eagerly flock to drugs that promise to do the same job—albeit that job might not even be needed. For although the lowering of cholesterol has never been shown to reduce the incidence of heart attacks, the public has become inured to the false idea that it will. The advice of many doctors notwithstanding, patients avidly demand anything that *might* lower cholesterol, especially a drug that will obviate the need for diet or exercise.

There are drugs that will lower blood cholesterol as measured by a laboratory test. But where does that "lowered" cholesterol go? In a few instances, it is possible to measure an increased amount of cholesterol coming out of the body; in other instances, it is just as possible to show an increased amount of cholesterol being deposited in the heart and other body organs as the blood cholesterol is reduced. And who is to say that this latter effect is good?

Because there will be many who will still insist on reducing their blood cholesterol levels, no matter what is said against the cholesterol-heart disease hypothesis, it seems only proper to discuss the drugs that work in this area.

Two things must be stipulated about the use of drugs to lower cholesterol. First, unlike the use of any "special" diet which can cause harm if carried to an extreme, the use of drugs are much easier to control. Some people will take an excess of drugs, as they would an excess of polyunsaturates, but there is less chance that an individual will risk the hazards of an overdose of this kind of drug. Moreover, the physician has some control over the amount of drugs a patient takes, since his prescription is necessary to obtain them. The side-effects of many drugs can also force an individual to limit the amount of medicine, over that prescribed, that he might take on his own.

Second, almost all of the drugs to lower cholesterol (called hypocholesteremic agents) are fairly new, and no one knows what the side-effects and toxic reactions will be after several years of use. In the past, most of these drugs have caused great harm. The dangers must be kept in mind, along with the knowledge that the drug is being taken for a purpose that has no scientific verification, to date.

As there are exceptions to all rules, there are exceptions in the use of hypocholesteremic drugs. If a physician can determine the exact cause of a high blood cholesterol, he can prescribe a drug that will work in that specific area. For example, if someone has an elevated cholesterol due to low thyroid activity, the mere balancing of thyroid function will reduce the cholesterol level. This balancing might be accomplished through the use of whole thyroid hormone, or through the use of a fraction of thyroid that has a lessened hyperactive effect on the whole body. This newest form of thyroid, called dextrothyroxine, has been shown to speed up the destruction of cholesterol and the end products of this destruction can actually be measured as they are excreted from the body. Because this drug still has some metabolic effect, it is not advised in all cases. It must be selectively prescribed by a physician who is aware of the patient's total metabolic state. And, there are patients whose cholesterol does not seem to respond at all to this particular drug.

Various vitamins have been shown to lower blood cholesterol, but these vitamins must be taken in very large amounts compared to what is usually prescribed. C and E are two such vitamins, but the one used longest to reduce blood cholesterol is niacin (nicotinic acid or vitamin B-3). So far, the exact way this vitamin works is not known, and, as with the special thyroid drug mentioned above, not all patients achieve a cholesterol lowering effect, no matter how much of the vitamin is given. Those who take large doses of niacin complain of an initial side-effect of severe flushing of the skin, fairly consistently described as the pins-and-needles itching similar to what one feels after having been in the sun too long. This reaction does seem to disappear if the patient can stay on the medicine for a week or so, and bear the constant redness and "burning" sensations of the skin, along with some nausea and stomach pains. Of interest, niacin is sometimes used in combination with other drugs as an aid in the treatment of certain mental and emotional problems. It is possible that its reported anxiety-reducing action could have some effect in cholesterol lowering. But, as with any drug, there are a number of side-effects that could be warning signs of an unusual sensitivity to this vitamin.

Just as a vitamin seems to have the additional ability to lower blood cholesterol levels, so does a commonly used antibiotic called neomycin. This drug, most often used to sterilize the bowel prior to surgery, or when there is a severe intestinal infection, also prevents the absorption of cholesterol in the intestine by reducing the normal bacteria that usually aid in this process.

Another drug used to lower cholesterol, albeit at this time the use of this particular medicine does not have the sanction of the FDA for its cholesterol-reducing effect, is cholestyramine. This drug is a chemical resin that combines with the bile acids and other products that eventually make cholesterol, and thereby prevents its formation—at least from the bile acids. Some research studies have shown, however, that the body responds to this interference by manufacturing much more cholesterol in different ways. In addition, for most people who have tried this drug as a hypocholesteremic agent (it is sold primarily for certain gall bladder problems), it is a most difficult substance to swallow and hold down (it must *never* be taken in dry form). Some people develop diarrhea, some develop rashes and some develop severe nutritional deficiencies. This drug has many other dangerous side-effects that can only be detected through repeated intricate medical examinations.

Probably the most commonly prescribed drug to lower cholesterol levels is a product called clofibrate. This drug is believed to act by inhibiting the production of cholesterol in the liver (although the exact way it works is still not definite). As with cholestyramine, this is a difficult substance for many people to hold down, especially during the first few days. Many other side-effects of clofibrate have been reported, such as hair loss, itching, skin rash and some adverse liver and blood reactions. The latest two side-effects to be reported consist of pain in the muscles, and there is some evidence that certain muscle tissue is damaged, and the formation of gall stones.

With any of these drugs, there is always the possibility of drug interactions, or the interference of one drug with some other drug being prescribed. This problem seems most frequent if a patient is taking anticoagulants, or with patients taking drugs for kidney or liver problems. Here again, only a physician can judge the value of a drug to lower cholesterol, and then take into account all the possible problems that could arise from the drug alone, or from its reaction with some other medicine that is being used.

Then, one must keep in mind that the most recent long-term studies reveal that even if the cholesterol is lowered through the use of drugs, there is no indication that there is a lessening of heart attack deaths. Remember that the government requires any drug manufacturer who tries to sell his product to lower cholesterol, to warn every physician that no one knows whether the use of the drug will have any effect on reducing heart disease. Furthermore, no one knows if the use of these drugs might have a detrimental effect on the patient. The government statement really speaks for itself: even if your cholesterol can be lowered, there is no evidence that this lowering will be good for you.

In considering the use of drugs to lower cholesterol, some of the disastrous past experiences in this area should be considered. Many years ago Dr. Jeremiah Stamler advocated that men take large doses of estrogens to lower their cholesterol levels, on the basis that women who had active ovaries seemed to have less heart disease. Not only has the active-ovary theory of protection against heart disease been disproved, but the feminizing effects of these female hormones caused worse side-effects in men than some of the side-effects of the newer drugs. Most men can face nausea, vomiting, and other stomach complaints more readily than they can enlarged breasts, loss of libido, and impotence.

Then, several years ago there was the drug called triparanol (the commercial name was MER/29) which acted somewhat analogously to clofibrate in that it interfered with the production of cholesterol in the body. Although this drug was cleared for use by the FDA, the havoc wrought as a consequence of its use was unbelievable. Men developed cataracts, baldness and impotence among other adverse side-effects. The story is briefly, but completely, told in a fascinating manner in the book *In the Name of Profit.* *

The profit in the manufacture and sale of drugs to lower cholesterol is enormous and will undoubtedly continue as long as the lowering of cholesterol continues to be pushed as a panacea, and until a truly effective means of preventing heart disease is discovered.

* Robert Heilbroner *et al, In the Name of Profit,* (New York: Doubleday, 1972).

CHAPTER 10

STRESS AND HEART DISEASE

FREDERICK L. JONES, JR., M.D. of Danville, Pennsylvania, who specializes in internal medicine, has written a fictitious series of letters as a medical article for physicians. He calls his piece on preventive medicine "Letters to Harvey." In these letters Dr. Jones attempts to demonstrate to his medical colleagues how too much attention to a minor or non-existent problem can cause a great deal of harm to a patient. Moreso, the letters show how lack of sensitivity to a person's feelings can be fatal.

June 16

Dear Harvey,

Alice is in a dither. Shall she pack the striped or the polka-dot bikini? I myself settled without hesitation on hiphugging surf-riders and a pair of bongos. Old friend, your invitation was irresistible! Do you really think Spray Beach can cope with three swinging septuagenarians in January?

We just returned from my 50th reunion at Kenmore, a pleasant affair made even more delightful by my shooting a 90 in the gold tournament, and our discovery that excellent martinis are still mixed at the Hamp.

Retirement has been much better than I anticipated. I still keep up connections with old friends at the office by doing consultative work two mornings a week. Perry lives nearby, and he has two teenage ballplayers who like to shag grandpop's flies. Alice and I get out to a good restaurant once a week or so—and you know my weakness for good cheescake!

A nagging backache (from a solid 5 iron shot last week?) has finally convinced me to have a checkup. I suppose we should do the same for our bodies as we do for our cars. So I am going to the Atwater-Marshall Clinic for one of those thorough physicals which are in vogue. They call it "health maintenance"—preventive (or is it preventative?) medicine.

I'll let you know how it goes.

Winston

September 21

Dear Harvey,

A note on hotel stationery isn't much, but I want to brief you on my day at Atwater-Marshall Clinic. Such efficiency, and everyone I saw was polite and friendly. They don't miss a thing here, I'm sure.

At 8 o'clock this morning, I filled out a long questionnaire covering everything from measles to bed-wetting. In quick order I had blood taken, drank some sugar water, had a chest x-ray, cardiogram and breathing tests, and had blood taken again. About 11 o'clock I saw my doctor (Kenmore '58!) who went over my forms and asked some more questions. I felt a bit embarassed, since the best I could come up with was the appendectomy I had in the service and a bout with the hives about 25 years ago.

My backache had disappeared two months ago, but I felt obligated to mention it too. After a thorough exam, my doctor ordered more studies—"no stone unturned about that back pain, etc." So I am scheduled for tests tomorrow morning: IVP, spinal series, sigmoidoscopy, and barium enema. I see him tomorrow afternoon for final reports which I anticipate will be good. In truth I have never felt better.

Alice surprised me tonight with a lovely meerschaum for my collection and a pound of John Cotton. At least I can have a good pipe in the morning, even if I do have to miss breakfast.

Winston

November 18

Dear Harvey,

These past two months have seen a great change in my life. I never thought much about my health before, but since my trip to the Clinic I seem to be devoting almost full time to it. Most of the tests were normal, but a few revealed unsuspected problems which demanded preventive measures.

First of all, I am a diabetic. My blood sugar tests were mildly but definitely abnormal, and the same was true of my cholesterol and uric acid. My cardiogram showed a few premature contractions and some changes that the doctor regarded as "nonspecific," but which might indicate coronary artery disease. The x-rays of my colon showed diverticulosis.

A therapeutic dietician instructed Alice and me in a special diet—diabetic, low fat, low cholesterol, low residue. Good-bye to those nights out for dinner and good-bye to the cheesecake. In fact, it has been good-bye to almost everything I enjoyed eating. No highball before supper. And the deepest cut of all, the doctor said I had to give up my pipe.

I am taking several drugs now: quinidine to stop the premature contractions, something to lower uric acid and a capsule to control my cholesterol. I test my urine for sugar every morning and go to our doctor for a blood sugar every month. So far I am doing well, he tells me. But somehow I don't feel the same.

The doctor at Atwater-Marshall told me to "take it easy," so I felt it best to give up my mornings at the office and reluctantly have confined my golf to a few turns on the putting green. Alice and I still look forward to visiting you this winter although I'm afraid I won't be a very sprightly guest.

Do you have a good internist in Spray Beach?

Winston

December 28

Dear Harvey,

I am indeed sorry that Alice and I will be unable to come to Spray Beach next month. May we have a rain check? I have been fatigued and irritable—I guess I miss that old tranquilizing pipe—

and have grown thin. Really, I would cut a rather poor figure on the strand. I sleep poorly, but hate to get up. I don't mind the pills since I've grown accustomed to them, and the diet isn't hard to follow. Actually I don't much care if I eat or not. My doctor can't find anything wrong, and I am following to the letter all the instructions of the Clinic.

Harvey, it's astonishing how everything can go to pieces all at once when you're 70. I can hardly believe I felt so well last summer.

Winston

March 8

Dear Harvey,

Win passed away on Wednesday. He was admitted to Cedars Hospital a week before with a case of flu which turned into pneumonia. At first they gave him an excellent chance to recover, but he just didn't seem to care. I don't believe he wanted to live.

Our doctor told me that before Win died his cardiogram, blood sugar, cholesterol and uric acid were all normal.

Alice

This series of letters illustrates what a strain any individual can be put under by pressures that seem to close in on him, frustrate him, and make life just not worth living.

A diet that makes a person miserable, makes him "heart-conscious," makes him worry that whatever he eats, or wants to eat, may give him a heart attack, may be defeating the very purpose of that diet. In treating the patient's physical body, but forgetting that the patient also has feelings, the well-meaning physician may be turning the patient into a stress-ridden heart-neurotic. Of course, stress is a relative and even subjective thing; what might easily upset one person could go completely unnoticed by another.

Emotional stress, or the way we react to life's situations, seems to cause more heart disease than do all other risk factors combined. If you eat excessively and are overweight, if you smoke a great deal or if you avoid any form of physical exercise, you may be contributing to the development of heart disease. But the most recent scientific evidence indicates that all of these factors put together are probably not as dangerous as the tension and anger that you allow to build up inside of you.

It is a proven medical fact that someone with diabetes has a far more difficult time with his disease if he becomes emotionally upset, no matter how much or how little sugar he eats. The same type of stress affects many other diseases, including heart disease. The way people respond to stressful situations is extremely important to their health and their hearts. More than 200 years ago, a famous physician, John Hunter, remarked in regard to heart disease that he felt his life was "in the hands of any rascal who chooses to annoy and tease me." Perhaps it is significant that he died suddenly only a few minutes after a violent argument during a board meeting at his hospital. And, as if to confirm Dr. Hunter's construct, the most recent studies by today's cardiologists show a greater incidence of heart disease among those whose attitudes toward their occupations or professions cause them the greatest amount of anxiety or tension.

Around 1900, Sir William Osler, sometimes considered the father of modern medicine, wrote: "in the worry and strain of modern life, arterial degeneration is not only very common but develops at a relatively early age. For this I believe that the high pressure at which men live and the habit of working the machine to its maximum capacity are responsible rather than excesses in eating and drinking."

As recently as December, 1971, a famous English physician, Dr. Stanley S. Gilder, wrote: "In the British medical press we get something new every month and the wonder is that the public still take notice of it all . . . should not the eager beavers be told that the atmosphere of anxiety they create also has a profound effect on health? In the last analysis it is anxiety that is the hidden destroyer of the contemporary world, not tobacco, nor coffee, nor soft water.

"Human survival depends on morale, as every military commander knows. So perhaps some of our research workers will pay a little attention to means of reducing anxiety rather than increasing it."

Physiologically, the harmful way stress works on the body can easily be demonstrated. Whenever there is stress, the adrenal glands produce an excess of several different hormones (one of these hormones, adrenalin, causes the heart to beat faster). At the same time, other adrenal substances cause the heart to need more oxygen which the body cannot always supply immediately. The faster, yet less effective, heart beat also decreases the amount of oxygen to both the heart and brain. The end result, hopefully temporary, is virtually identical to the loss of oxygen that is caused by an actual heart attack. Some other adrenal products make the body much more susceptible to infection, and this could explain the "virus theory" of heart disease.

Of special interest to those who live in fear of heart disease is the work of Dr. Meyer Friedman of San Francisco. He has demonstrated (in addition to his work to show that the type of fat one eats has no real effect on the blood circulation or blood cholesterol level) that a particular, easily identifiable, personality type is more prone to heart disease than other types. Dr. Friedman calls this personality "Type A." And he now believes that this behavior pattern is a cause of heart disease and not merely a contributory or associated factor. To quote Dr. Friedman: "Type A behavior pattern is the most important factor in precipitating adult coronary heart disease in this country." He also says that this factor "may be so potent in its lethalness that it quite dwarfs the possible harmfulness of the American diet." Interestingly, it has been shown that the administration of steroid hormones, which are the same as those produced by the adrenals when a person is under stress, can cause a Type A personality in someone receiving that drug.

What is Type A behavior? While comprised of many different personality characteristics, the one most prominent thing about a Type A man is his urgency about time. He strives to be absolutely punctual, no matter what the cost in emotional strain. What is even worse, he becomes severely aggravated by anyone who keeps him waiting, even if it honestly cannot be helped. Such an attitude is not limited to his work, but may come to the surface if a waiter in a restaurant simply "seems" slower than expected. If someone delays the start of a meeting, even a social one with no great business importance, or if the Type A man "feels" an automobile is traveling too slowly in his traffic lane, he is far more disturbed than the average person. Ambition alone does not have any deleterious effects on the heart or body, but this man is ambitious and competitive to an extreme. The Type A personality is in evidence when the aggressive pursuit of the appearance of success is coupled with irritation at anything or anyone that is conceived to slow down or interfere with that success.

There are many other ways to identify a Type A man. He is the one whose wife is constantly telling him to "take it easy," or "slow down." He is constantly interrupting the person who is talking to him and attempts to finish the sentence for him.

What is most paradoxical about this man striving so hard to accomplish something—anything—is that his counterpart, called a "Type B" personality, is almost always more successful, no matter what the type of work being done. The Type B man is more creative and does not let time influence his judgments. He is calmer and yet at the same time expresses more appropriate emotional responses to situations. The Type A man, for example, rarely admits to worry or fear. He denies he is ever "bothered" about things, while the Type B man does not hesitate to reflect his emotions—especially those that are positive, such as love and affection.

Dr. Friedman's classification of the Type A personality is based on studying more than 3500 subjects in such minute detail that even speech patterns were recorded. It was discovered that Type A has a tendency to speak frequently, rapidly and explosively, and was also given to sudden gestures such as fist-clenching, desk pounding and taut facial grimaces. But the most pervasive characteristic of the Type A seems to be his preoccupation with competitiveness, often without any obvious goal in mind—competition simply for competition's sake.

Dr. Friedman believes that the Type A personality is far more at risk of a heart attack right after eating a meal, regardless of the type or amount of fat eaten. Eating increases the circulation of blood to the intestines to about four times what it usually is, so that if there is any stress imposed at this time, and the circulation to the heart is already markedly decreased, the chances for sudden heart stoppage increase to an extreme.

In another study of the relation of stress to heart disease, the emotional make-up of patients with known heart disease was investigated. It was found that more than four times as many people in hospitals with heart problems had experienced some acute emotional conflict they could not handle within three days prior to their hospitalization. The most common conflict was a violent argument in which the Type A personality did not feel he won, although, at the time, such a defeat was not admitted either inwardly or outwardly.

Another, somewhat similar study of Eastman Kodak workers who died suddenly from heart attacks, although they had been in apparent good physical health to the moment of the attack, revealed that psychological factors were most likely the cause of death. Of 26 employees studied in retrospect, almost all of them had been "running sad" just prior to their fatal episode. After the fact, it was admitted by both wives and friends that these men had been quite depressed, and it was also recalled that some sudden, very unpleasant development occurred just before the heart attack. In a parallel study at the same company, the physician who made the initial observation then went on to study men who had had heart attacks but who had survived. The psychological data obtained in this way, which was not second-hand, confirmed the psychosocial conditions that are quite evidently a major cause of heart disease.

A study of patients who were admitted to a hospital for heart attacks and were treated for their psychological stress as well as for their heart disease, had their mortality reduced 75 percent. Uncontrolled or unexpressed emotions, which manifest themselves as impatient or the unwillingness to face a challenge rationally, are great precipitating factors in heart disease, and, unfortunately, the diet that can control emotions has yet to be discovered.

Stress was recognized as a significant risk factor in heart disease in a recent report by the National Heart and Lung Institute Task Force on Arteriosclerosis which stated: "Epidemiologic studies have shown that persons who undergo a major change in their cultural environment have increased risk of coronary disease. These changes, termed social mobility, include moving to a new nation, from a farm to the city, changing one's career or one's social status. A related group having increased coronary risk are those persons experiencing status incongruity. By this is meant the situation where different social characteristics of a person simultaneously place him at different levels of the social hierarchy. Social scientists hypothesize that both social mobility and status incongruity are likely to increase feelings of personal insecurity and hence produce 'stress'."

The report goes on to say: "Several studies report that coronary events have often been preceded by some type of severe personal loss, such as death of a loved one, loss of a job, financial reversal, or loss of self-esteem such as occasioned by the breakup of a love relationship. Other workers implicate work overload, including long hours of overtime work or increasing burdens of job responsibility, as temporal antecedents to the emergence of coronary disease."

A cardiologist, James S. Haimsohn M.D., of Memphis says: "emotional stress and strain is the major factor among the many factors producing heart attacks. Heart attacks can be brought on by an acute emotionally traumatic experience or by long term frustration."

Dr. Ingvar Liljefors, of Sweden, has shown that heart disease is closely linked to a person's *attitude* toward his work, rather than the work itself. While Dr. Liljefors could find absolutely no relationship between heart disease and how much fat a person ate, he did find far more heart disease in those whose ambition to exert authority was so all consuming that it displaced all else in the struggle for a prominent position on the social scale.

Dr. Reuben E. Kron, of the University of Pennsylvania, notes that several different researchers have indicated that emotional stress may precipitate a heart attack. He feels: "there is increasing evidence that atherosclerosis alone cannot adequately explain the occurrence of most vascular disease attributed to it." Dr. Kron's own studies show that psychological stress can cause a heart attack by altering the viscosity of the blood.

Dr. Henry I. Russek of New York, has written: ". . . even the statistical relationship between smoking and coronary disease may reflect the importance of emotional stress rather than cigarettes themselves."

A 1971 report by the World Health Organization on "Society, Stress, and Disease," indicated that the serenity of daily life in Roseto, Pennsylvania was the real reason for the virtual absence of heart attacks there, in spite of the fact that the people ate an excessive amount of saturated fats, were overweight, and smoked. Some of the particular observations on the social life of Roseto included the fact that the men were the unchallenged heads of their households, everyone had great civic pride and, most of all, there was mutual support and understanding throughout the entire community.

Dr. Hans Selye, who is considered the originator of today's stress theory in relation to disease, states that "emotional tension is the most common human stressor agent." When he reproduces in animals the hormone situation that parallels stress in humans, he notes that many animals succumb to an acute cardiac death. When he added a polyunsaturated fat to the animal's diet while inducing stress, the incidence of death from heart disease rises to one hundred percent. When the animals are fed meat fats, however, the death rate is almost halved, even with the stressful situation.

With so much formidable evidence to the contrary, the American Heart Association continues to derogate stress as a factor in heart disease while reaffirming diet and cholesterol as the major culprits. Paradoxically, the Association admits that an emotional upset increases the work of the heart. However, the American Heart Association refrains from comment about the effect of stress on people who already have an impaired heart. It even goes so far in trying to disparage the stress theory as to state that the disagreeable symptoms that come from emotional tension, such as palpitation, weakness, faintness, etc., are usually harmless.

The rules and restriction imposed by government as well as some of those agencies, industries, and the media who hold themselves forth as experts in what is best for the masses, totally ignore the individual and his needs. Their aim seems to be to reduce people to the level of sheep in robbing them of self-determination and the right to be unique. The individual was not created to have an official mind make so small a decision for him as to whether he should smoke, drink or eat eggs for breakfast.

Large organizations, the media, voluntary health agencies and government agencies too often try to usurp the individual's right to think for himself, to follow the truth as he sees it. They create and support fear for commercial purposes. These and the many other pressures that the individual is subject to every day of his life, rob him of his equanimity, his joy in living, the effects of which diet certainly cannot remedy.

Dr. William Kitchiner wrote in 1817: ". . . for the Stomach is the mainspring of our System—if it be not sufficiently wound up to warm the Heart and support the Circulation, the whole business of Life will, in proportion, be ineffectively performed." There are those today who may not agree that the stomach is the mainspring of our system, but there is no doubt that mealtime should be a time of pleasure with tension reduced as much as possible.

If fear for your heart causes stress, then by all means follow a diet that will eliminate that stress. If a special "heart-conscious" diet that restricts meat protein and forces fish makes you miserable, by all means eat meat, if possible just a little less and with the fat cut off, and you will probably do yourself more good than following the diet that distressed you.

"All right," you say, "I accept that stress plays a large part in heart disease. What can I do about it? Some problems just won't go away."

The best, and yet the most annoying piece of advice ever given is, "Don't worry." Unless someone can solve the problems that make you worry, there is no way to stop worrying on command. The responsibilities, the need for decisions, the frustrations and fears that cause anxiety are never easy to eliminate. Some of them are life-long companions. While there may be no easy answer to the problems that give you stress, there are ways of dealing with that stress that can ameliorate it and make it less painful or dangerous to the physical functioning of your body.

Several physicians suggest wine with meals as a means of releasing tension. A pre-dinner aperitif may serve the same purpose. A moderate amount of alcohol is still considered by many as less harmful than tranquilizers. An occasional smoke may prove soothing. But this does not mean regular heavy smoking or drinking. Anyone addicted to alcohol, cigarettes or drugs is trying to commit suicide anyway, so why should he worry about heart disease?

Sports are often great temporary distractors from one's worries. A good swim, a game of tennis or even a long walk can reduce tension and prove very refreshing. A shopping spree or pouring one's heart out to an understanding friend can have the same effect. Sex, too, has often been said to be a great releaser of tensions. Perhaps this is why married people are statistically healthier than single people. Concerning the relationship of love to disease, Dr. John C. Cassel of the University of North Carolina School of Public Health believes that the lack of warm social approval can result in marked alterations in hormone levels and nervous system changes. He said: "If there is no such thing, I'd find it hard to explain why divorced men have a death rate three to five times higher than married men of the same age."

Professional help may be necessary in extreme cases of emotional stress where the patient is unable or unwilling to cope.

A substantial part of relieving stress or anxiety is in "unwinding." As with diet, this is not a simple task for most people. But, under the supervision of a family physician, the right tranquilizer can be found to offer temporary relief of acute stress. Why the "right" tranquilizer? Because each individual reacts differently. Where a particular drug offers an easing of tension for one person, that same medicine could make another person drowsy or it could even make an emotional crisis appear far worse than it is. Some people suffer from a dry mouth or blurring of their vision on the smallest dose of one drug, while another chemically different preparation could induce relaxation without any disturbing side-effects. Some tranquilizers are so strong they can cause blood changes, and must be taken only with constant professional vigilance. And, keep in mind that some anti-histamine drugs do more for one's anxiety than they do for one's allergy.

Generally speaking, the best tranquilizer is the one with which your own doctor has had the most experience. The most effective, when properly used, however, are still the barbiturates, with butabarbital the one that seems the most gentle in its action and the least irritating when it wears off. Anti-depressant drugs are probably the strongest of the lot and carry with them the greatest incidence of dangerous side-effects—if, and when, used improperly.

The use of a medicine to help one through a stressful crisis is only a stop-gap measure. When tranquilizers become a crutch, a habitual thing, the search for a solution to the cause of chronic emotional stress may never even begin. For some people it is easier just to go on benumbed. They do not realize that they are on the primrose path to dependency, where eventually the tension caused by the constant need for pills will override the stress for which the pills were prescribed. But in moments of acute anxiety it does seem much more sensible to relieve the acute stress rather than subject the heart and blood vessels to all of the secondary effects the hormones and body chemicals of anxiety produce.

In chronic stress, healthier ways of reacting can be established if there is a conscientious desire to do so. Energies can be channeled so that they are not wasted in useless fretting, anxiety and hostility. Time does not have to be the master. Setting a meaningful goal and working toward that goal, rather than exhausting energy in meaningless competitions will eliminate some of the stress that the Type A personality suffers. The person who can "slow down" even a little will markedly decrease his risks for all illness, including heart disease.

Even the *Journal of the American Medical Association* recently recognized the deleterious or stressful reactions that can be caused in the patient when the doctor deprives him of pleasure.

> Much has been written in the medical literature about pain, but little about pleasure. This is understandable. After all, it is pain, not pleasure that brings the patient to the doctor. Still, the physician is very much involved with pleasure. In fact, while engaged in a hot war against pain he has been fighting all along a cold war against many pleasures—drink, tobacco, food, drugs, lust, and leisure. . . . Even if we do not fully accept Voltaire's dictum that 'pleasure is the object, the duty, and the goal of all rational creatures,' we must give it important consideration when assessing the need for proscribing pleasure.

One physician, Dr. Mark D. Altschule, professor of medicine at Harvard, has often expressed his awareness of, and sensitivity toward, a patient's needs beyond the physical. In regard to the pressures being put on everyone to go on low cholesterol, high polyunsaturate diets, he wrote: "Low cholesterol cooking changes what should be a simple pleasure, *i.e.,* eating, to a complicated emotional experience in which the cook is in a constant state of resentment (wondering 'O Lord, what next?'), the diners are bored by a monotonous diet, and the patient is terrified by the possibility that his low fat intake is not low enough to save his life."

Dr. Altschule's recommendation to physicians concerning the cholesterol controversy was: "Ten centuries ago extreme abstemiousness was believed to be a way of enriching life after death. Today marked abstemiousness with respect to dietary fat is regarded by some as a way of prolonging life on earth. There is no reason to believe that mortifying the flesh in this way will accomplish either aim. If any of the cardinal sins does prove to be specifically implicated in atherogenesis it is more likely to be sloth [and stress] than gluttony."

ANNOTATED BIBLIOGRAPHY
AND DOCUMENTATION

ANNOTATED BIBLIOGRAPHY
AND DOCUMENTATION

In addition to the many specific, supportive, references in the main part of the book, there are hundreds of other published medical articles, reports of scientific papers that have been given at medical and nutrition meetings, and reports of research on the relationship of cholesterol to heart disease. All have concluded that there is no connection between reducing the laboratory-measured blood cholesterol—be it by any special diet—and the lessening of heart attacks. For those who wish to pursue any, or all, of the many aspects of the cholesterol controversy in detail, corroborative documentation follows. The medical journals that are cited may be found in a county medical society library, a medical school library, or in most large hospital libraries. Wherever possible, a journalist's report on the medical research is given, rather than the original technical presentation, in order to make the reading easier. At the end of this bibliography are the addresses where most of the medical news publications may be obtained.

1. LET THE CONSUMER BE WARY

The attitude of the federal government is clearly shown by its public statement:

U. S. DEPARTMENT OF
HEALTH, EDUCATION, AND WELFARE

Food and Drug Administration
Washington 25, D. C.

FOR RELEASE IN P.M. PAPERS
Wednesday, May 27, 1964

The Food and Drug Administration, U. S. Department of Health, Education, and Welfare, today said that legal action will be taken if vegetable oil products continue to be misbranded with claims that they are "poly-unsaturated" and thus supposedly effective in treating or preventing heart or artery disease.

George P. Larrick, Commissioner of Food and Drugs, made the announcement at a meeting of FDA's Public Service Committee, composed of representatives of national consumer organizations.

Mr. Larrick told the consumer representatives that FDA's decision to proceed against the health claims being made for vegetable oil products was based on the results of a consumer survey on public understanding of current labeling of such products. He said the survey shows that label terms such as "polyunsaturated," "unsaturated," "low in cholesterol," and similar statements mislead many people to believe that these foods will reduce blood cholesterol and thus be effective in treating or preventing heart and artery diseases. Other misleading phrases include, "ask your doctor," "better for people's health," "are you concerned about saturated fats," and "better for you because it's made from 100% golden corn oil."

The Commissioner urged the food industry to correct promptly such labeling and promotional practices for oils, fats and related foods which tend to mislead consumers.

The consumer survey, made under contract by A.R.S. Surveys, Division of CEIR, Inc., New York City, consisted of 780 personal interviews during May and June, 1963, with individuals statistically chosen to be representative of the adult population in households throughout the United States. Interviews were conducted in 30 metropolitan and nonmetropolitan areas.

Commissioner Larrick said that in the light of the survey results, "the Food and Drug Administration reaffirms its official Statement of Policy of December 10, 1959." The policy statement said any claim, whether direct or implied, in the labeling of fats and oils or other fatty substances offered to the general public that such foods will prevent, mitigate or cure heart or artery diseases, is false and misleading and is considered a misbranding under Federal law.

At that time FDA pointed out that the role of cholesterol in heart and artery diseases had not been scientifically established and that a causal relationship between blood cholesterol levels and these diseases had not been proved. FDA today said that although scientific investigations since 1959 have contributed materially to knowledge of fat metabolism, the role of fats in artery and heart disease remains unresolved.

Commissioner Larrick made the following statement:

"Scientific investigations of fatty substances as a possible factor in lowering blood cholesterol and of the role of blood cholesterol in affecting heart and artery diseases should be continued. The 1959 policy statement did not and does not interfere in any way with legitimate research and clinical evaluation of unsaturated fats in the diet. What the policy statement is intended to do is prevent the promotion of foods to the lay public for their use without medical supervision in attempting to reduce blood cholesterol.

"The public has been misled into believing that foods labeled as 'polyunsaturated,' 'low (or lower) in cholesterol' or 'made from 100% golden corn oil' can be used as simple measures, without other dietary changes, to so affect blood cholesterol as to prevent or treat heart and artery disease. Such foods play no significant part in reducing blood cholesterol unless the diet is changed drastically in other respects. Even when blood cholesterol levels are lowered under careful medical supervision the significance of such lowering in the prevention and treatment of heart and artery disease has not been established and is still experimental."

Mr. Larrick urged that any promotion of products that purport to be of value for cholesterol reduction be directed solely to the medical profession. He said that a lay person is neither able to determine for himself what practices, if any, should be followed in controlling the cholesterol level of the blood, nor to put dietary changes into effect with assurance that the intended objectives will be obtained.

Whether or not dietary changes are needed in the treatment or prevention of heart and artery disease can be determined only by a physician, after making suitable tests," Mr. Larrick said.

To learn how certain health groups have specifically misled the public on cholesterol through the manipulation of statistics, see the chapter "On Inferring Causality from Observed Observations," by Dr. J. Yerushalmy of the University of California School of Public Health, Berkeley, in the book *Controversies in Internal Medicine,* edited by Inglefinger. Philadelphia: W. B. Saunders, 1966. In the same book there is another chapter "The Uselessness of Diet in the Treatment of Atherosclerosis," by Mark

D. Altschule, M.D., professor of medicine at Harvard University. Dr. Altschule has more recently affirmed his medical judgement in an article, "Can Diet Prevent Atherogenesis? If so, what Diet?" in the scientific journal *Medical Counterpoint* (November, 1970).

Because the "Framingham Study" is referred to so often as a basis for the alleged cholesterol-diet-heart disease relationship, a transcript of the "Meet the Press" program for April 23, 1972, (available for 10 cents and a stamped, self-addressed envelope from Merkle Press, Inc., Box 2111, Washington, D.C. 20013) will reveal that Dr. J. Willis Hurst, president of the American Heart Association (and former President Johnson's personal physician) has publicly stated that in the Framingham Study there was no real testing for, nor any relationship to, what a person eats and his blood cholesterol levels, nor was there any evidence that lowering the blood cholesterol level will have any effect in protecting against a heart attack. There are many eminent cardiologists, one such individual being Dr. Louis N. Katz, director emeritus of the Cardiovascular Institute, Michael Reese Hospital and Medical Center in Chicago, who has said that in the matter of preventing and/or treating heart disease: "Scientific proof of the value of diet is still lacking" (*Internal Medicine News*, June 1, 1971).

Where the relationship of heart disease to diet and to blood cholesterol levels has been objectively studied for several years, the concensus is that " 'high' plasma cholesterol levels do not indicate any certainty of coronary heart disease." (Report of a Committee of the Royal Society of New Zealand, 1971, available for $3.00 from: General Secretary, The Royal Society of New Zealand, P. O. Box 196, Wellington, N.Z.) *The Medical Journal of Australia* in two different issues (July 24, p. 219, and July 31, p. 282, 1971) has also published evidence against any relationship between diet and heart disease. Dr. Michael DeBakey, of Baylor College of Medicine, has studied 1,700 patients who had definite, severe, atherosclerosis and found 80 percent of these patients had *normal* blood cholesterol levels. Dr. DeBakey has stated he sees no relationship between diet, cholesterol and heart disease. He is quoted: "It just doesn't make sense that elevated cholesterol levels are the cause of coronary artery disease" (in a lecture before the Danciger Institute of Menorah Medical Center, Kansas City, Missouri, in 1971).

For some easy to read reports on the most recent evidence to show there is no relationship between what you eat (in the matter of polyunsaturates) and heart disease, see *Medical World News* for August 28, and September 11, 1970.

Although there are numerous references throughout this book to show the absolute lack of any relationship between diet, cholesterol and the prevention and/or treatment of heart disease, in his lecture before the American College of Physicians, Dr. Lars Werkö, of Göteborb, Sweden concluded that "Despite considerable effort nobody has been able to demonstrate that it is possible to reduce the incidence of ischemic [lack of oxygen] heart disease by lowering serum cholesterol." ("Can We Prevent Heart Disease?" *Annals of Internal Medicine*, 74:278, February, 1971).

Not that ample research specifically on this hypothesis has not been performed. In England a very carefully controlled study was made to see if a special diet to lower blood cholesterol would, in fact, prevent heart disease. After six years, not only did the special diet have no real effect on a patient's cholesterol—and this diet went to the extreme in enforcing polyunsaturates—but the ultimate conclusion was that "There is no evidence from the London trial that the relapse-rate in myocardial infarction [heart attack] is materially affected by the unsaturated fat content of the diet used" (*Lancet, 2*:693, September 28, 1968). Continuing with this same conclusion, *The Medical Letter* (May 15, 1970) has told physicians: "It is still not certain that elevation of blood lipids [cholesterol is a lipid] is a major contributing cause of atherosclerosis and ischemic vascular disease; nor that reduction of lipid levels by diet or drugs helps prevent the development or progression of ischemic vascular disease." In a more recent issue of *The Medical Letter* (July 9, 1971), the previous pronouncement was sustained: "There is no conclusive evidence that diets low in saturated fats or cholesterol help control atheroma and arteriosclerotic complications."

The report by the Agricultural Research Service to the U.S. Senate that corn oil causes more cholesterol than dairy products or meat fats may be obtained from the office of Senator George D. Aiken, Washington, D.C. 20510. Dr. Caster's similar research was presented to the American Institute of Nutrition meeting in Atlantic City in 1972. It may be found in *Federation Proceedings* (FASEB), *31*:674A, 1972.

Dr. George V. Mann's comments on the complicity of certain food manufacturers and health agencies will be found in *Medical World News* for January 8, 1971 and August 18, 1972.

But in spite of the illegality of advertising and promoting polyunsaturated fats as a direct means to prevent and treat heart disease, as seen in newspapers, magazines and on TV, the commercial pressure on the consumer persists. And it is precisely because of such pressure that so many other possible causes of heart disease go inadequately researched. While this book is not intended to discuss the non-cholesterol related allegations for heart troubles, there are other approaches to preventing heart attacks that deserve intensive study but which are virtually ignored because most government and commercial grants tend to obscure new, and different, research ideas. As an example, George E. Burch, M.D., chairman of the department of medicine at Tulane University, has proposed, with ample supporting evidence, a virus infection theory of heart and artery disease—with no relationship to diet whatsoever. Dr. Burch, citing his own research in which he caused damage to the heart and arteries of animals through deliberate infection with a virus (and also compared this with the heart and artery disease that comes from a syphilis infection), proposes that virus infections in childhood may well be the precipitating factor that causes artery damage in later years (Presented at the December, 1971, meeting of the American Medical Association). At the same time, Dr. Sidney E. Grossberg, of the Medical College of Wisconsin, has shown that certain virus infections also cause changes in blood cholesterol levels (*Medical World News,* September 24, 1971).

Some new work has been done to show either the value or destructiveness of trace elements (certain minerals such as chromium, cadmium, zinc, selenium, etc.) in relation to heart disease (*Roche Image of Medicine and Research,* March, 1972). Where cadmium increases in the diet, there seems to be a greater amount of heart disease deaths (*Medical Tribune,* June 14, 1972). The softness of water, which depends on its mineral content, has been linked to sudden death from heart disease (*American Journal of Epidemiology, 92:*90, August, 1970). And some of the chemicals in the air, ones that become excessive when there is smog, can cause damage to the blood vessels—especially if one eats a large amount of polyunsaturated fats (*Archives of Environmental Health,* 22:32, January, 1971).

Details of how carbon monoxide is linked to heart disease are in *The Journal of the American Medical Association,* 221:456, July 31, 1972.

Very little work is being done on the relationship of genetics to heart disease. This aspect of an inherited tendency to heart attack seems much more important, and useful, than some specific, unproved diet. For example, a study by Dr. Michel Ibrahim, of the University of North Carolina, showed that girls are much more likely to develop heart disease if their fathers have had heart trouble (Presented at the 1971 meeting of the American Public Health Association). In another, somewhat related, study of more than 2,600 relatives of heart attack victims, it was found that at least 20 percent had a genetically transmitted form of the disease—completely different from familial hypercholesteremia which also exists (Presented to the 1972 meeting of the Association of American Physicians by Dr. Joseph L. Goldstein of the University of Washington). Even the blood type you inherit may have an influence on future heart troubles. Those with Type A blood seem more prone to heart disease (*Internal Medicine Digest,* September, 1970, abstracting an article from *Lancet,* one of England's major medical journals; *Modern Medicine,* September 6, 1971).

One of the newest theories to explain the sudden rise in heart disease in this century is that of Kurt A. Oster, M.D., of Bridgeport, Conn., who feels that the homogenization of milk breaks down the normal-sized fat particles and allows an enzyme called xanthine oxidase to enter the blood stream which, in turn, destroys vital body chemicals that would normally protect the arteries of the heart. To back up his idea, Dr. Oster claims that the death rate from heart disease in different countries is proportionate to how much homogenized milk people drink, and also is far less in countries where the people normally boil their milk before drinking—which destroys the xanthine oxidase ("Role of Plasmalogen in Heart Disease," in *Myocardiology,* Volume I, Baltimore: University Park Press, 1972).

In truth, there is a lack of "predictors" that would indicate a future heart attack (Dr. R. Foster Scott, of Albany, N.Y., in a report to the American Heart Association in 1971). And, in a very comprehensive study to determine clues to an imminent heart attack, Dr. Mary Fulton of Edinburgh, Scotland, came up with "unstable angina" (irregular chest pains with no definite pattern of time or intensity) as "the best existing *short-time* predictor." Seventy-one additional doctors worked with Dr. Fulton, and the total number of patients under study was 25,000. But even here, if there was no heart attack within four weeks after the chest pains, there was no real predictability (reported in *Lancet,* issue number 7756).

If you have any doubts that commercialism has been the chief factor in altering the American diet to the point where people do believe that an excess of polyunsaturates will prevent and treat heart disease—irrespective of existing laws that forbid such unproved health claims—there are many careful studies that show how the regular use of butter has decreased from 70 percent to only 25 percent; polyunsaturates have increased as regular family fare for 30 percent of the population, when it used to be a staple for only 4 percent. ("Trends in Fat Disappearance in the United States, 1909-1965 (*Journal of Nutrition, 93:*1, December, 1967). This observation is supported by the U.S. Department of Agriculture's Economic Report No. 138, issued in 1969, which shows the decrease in the use of all dairy foods. In 1971, the Agriculture Department's Report No. 136 adds that not only is the use of dairy food still decreasing, but eggs, too, are disappearing from the family table. The Special Survey Branch of the Agriculture Department concluded, in April, 1971, that the marked change in the type of fats people use came about strictly for heart-health purposes; people have been sufficiently brainwashed to think that polyunsaturated fats will help their hearts in spite of the fact there is absolutely no scientific evidence to back up this commercially promoted claim.

In a story about the present-day conflict between butter and margarine, food writer Dorothy Brown (the Philadelphia *Evening Bulletin,* August 16, 1972) reports that two-thirds of all Americans now use margarine instead of butter. Where once the deciding factor between the two spreads was price, Miss Brown cites the Department of Agriculture as saying: "today it's also fear of heart disease." In the article Dr. David Kritchevsky, professor of biochemistry at the University of Pennsylvania, makes a plea for all margarine labels to carry the same *warning* that is required for drugs used to lower cholesterol (see Chapter II).

While *The Journal of the American Medical Association* (*217:* 1238, August 30, 1971), reports that the American public is now "hip" to the atherogenic potential of saturated vs. polyunsaturated fats, a detailed study on the relationship of retail market food supplies (a reflection of what people buy) shows that while the sale of polyunsaturate to saturated fat ratio has increased more than 37 percent in the past 60 years, the amount of heart disease has not decreased; rather it has increased, leading to the conclusion that polyunsaturates do not lessen heart disease (*American Journal of Clinical Nutrition, 14:*169, March, 1964). Dr. Harold Kahn of the National Heart and Lung Institute reported in that same journal (*23:*879, July, 1970) that while polyunsaturates have more than doubled in the typical American diet, the levels of blood cholesterol have not really changed at all over the same period of time. Yet, he says, heart disease has increased which means there is no relationship to diet changes insofar as heart disease is concerned.

2. PITFALLS OF MEASURING

YOUR BLOOD CHOLESTEROL

To learn just how bad most laboratory testing really is, write to the Laboratory Division of the United States Center for Disease Control (Atlanta, Georgia 30333), and request a copy of its most recent survey of the accuracy of laboratories throughout the country. Inaccuracies in measuring cholesterol are quite common, but even when inept laboratories are discovered, the government rarely takes any action against those who do a sloppy job. Then, to understand the marked variation as to what is supposed to be a normal cholesterol level in the blood, simply ask the various laboratories in your area. In Los Angeles, 12 different laboratories came up with 12 different values with a discrepancy spread of more than 100.

As to how the blood cholesterol level fails to reflect disease within the body can best be demonstrated by people who have xanthelasma (the small, yellow, fatty deposit in the skin, most common on the eyelid but also on the elbow and over other body tendons). While most medical reports say that any xanthomatous plaque means high blood cholesterol levels, in fact more than half of the people who have such a lesion have a normal, or low, blood cholesterol (*Diseases of the Skin,* Philadelphia: W. B. Saunders Co.).

Dr. George Kozak, professor at Harvard Medical School has also found xanthomatous plaques in only half of his patients who have high blood cholesterols. He particularly noted that even if you do lower the cholesterol levels, you do *not* get rid of the yellow spots on the eyelids (*Hospital Medicine,* August, 1972).

Some newer research indicates that even a 14 hour fast, prior to measuring your blood cholesterol is not enough, especially if you have eaten a great deal of carbohydrates (*not* fats) the previous day or two. More than half of such people tested showed a temporarily high cholesterol reading (*Internal Medicine News,* June 1, 1972). Dr. Peter Kuo, of the University of Pennsylvania, feels that sugar alone will cause an extremely high cholesterol, with no evident relationship to heart disease (*Medical World News,* February 12, 1971).

Dr. Myron E. Tract, professor of pathology at Columbia University College of Physicians and Surgeons has compiled a list of commonly used drugs that will cause false results when blood cholesterol is measured (*Consultant,* September, 1972). Twenty-six out of 49 drugs studied altered the cholesterol level sufficiently to yield an error in the test results.

Although many medical laboratories advertise that through the use of tests such as cholesterol it is possible to prognosticate heart disease (*e.g., Laboratory Aids in Coronary Artery Disease and Myocardial Infarction,* published by Bio-Science Laboratories), the author of the booklet cited states: "The question of whether 'cholesterol is a known etiological factor in coronary disease' is so widely debated, and so subject to different interpretation that neither I nor anyone else can specifically claim it to be true at this time."

Various hormones, whether produced naturally by the body or taken as medicines, will severely alter one's blood cholesterol without causing heart disease. If one takes any cortisone product (and there are nearly 100 different variations of this steroid drug), the blood cholesterol will go way up. This has been noticed especially in patients who are treated for rheumatic disease (*Medical World News,* August 6, 1971). An increase in the amount of insulin in the body will also cause a concurrent elevated blood cholesterol (*Medical Tribune,* June 16, 1971; *Cardiology Abstracts,* September, 1968).

As has been mentioned, heredity seems to be a major cause of a high blood cholesterol—not necessarily related to a risk of heart disease, however. Dr. Sheila C. Mitchell, of the National Heart and Lung Institute, feels that until proved otherwise, an elevated cholesterol is always familial (presented to the 1972 meeting of the American College of Cardiology).

How exercise has an effect on one's cholesterol level is reported in the *New England Journal of Medicine, 279:*1001, October 31, 1968, as well as in *Modern Medicine,* June 14, 1971. Incidentally, Chuck Hughes, the professional football player who died of a heart attack during a game one Sunday, had a normal cholesterol level (*Medical World News,* November 12, 1971).

Animals exposed to severe, protracted, cold have high cholesterol levels, compared to similar animals exposed to moderate temperatures, but those with the elevated cholesterol have no sign of any heart disease (*Medical Counterpoint,* March, 1972).

That blood cholesterol levels can vary by the hour has been shown by John E. Peterson, M.D. (*Circulation, 22:*247, August, 1960). Dr. Peterson also showed an even greater variation when the subjects were exposed to various stresses—both physical and psychological. Psychological stress, however, seems to have the most marked influence on one's cholesterol levels. Two U.S. Navy experiments showed a profound rise in blood cholesterol whenever the individual was depressed or showed anger or fear (*Psychosomatic Medicine, 33:*399, September/October, 1971). The same relationship was found when the subjects expressed an unpleasant affect (state of mind) (*Archives of General Psychiatry, 26:*357, April, 1972). When medical students were subjected to extreme stressful situations, Dr. Vincent P. Carroll, Jr., of Los Angeles, found that cholesterol levels were extremely sensitive to the psychological stimuli (presented to the 1971 meeting of the American Heart Association).

At a U. S. Air Force base, it was found that cholesterol levels more than doubled when a patient underwent any severe emotional stress such as frustration (*American Journal of the Medical Sciences,* p. 133, February, 1960). And the relationship of occupational stress to the elevated blood cholesterol was clearly shown by Dr. Meyer Friedman (*Circulation, 22:*852, May, 1958). It was Dr. Friedman who also showed that individuals with a particular personality he calls "Type A" (who *always* put themselves under some form of pressure) had much higher cholesterol levels after eating no matter what type of fat they ate—even when the fat was polyunsaturated (*Circulation, 29:*874 June, 1964).

Some of Dr. Rose's work on how psychological stress will modify the cholesterol level can be found in the book *"Myocardiology - Recent Advances in Studies on Cardiac Structure and Metabolism,"* Baltimore: University Park Press, 1972. A great many more scientific references to stress and its effect on the body will be found in Chapter 10 of this book, and the bibliography for that chapter.

There is one more fact that should be mentioned here. That is the relationship of one's cholesterol level *after* having had heart disease. While it does appear that subsequent to heart troubles, a person's cholesterol level does go up, there is still no real relationship between heart disease and blood cholesterol (*American Journal of Clinical Nutrition, 23:* 178, February, 1970). And in a follow-up study of nearly 300 men who had heart disease for 20 years, it was reported: "There was no significant relationship between the serum cholesterol level and the incidence of soft criteria coronary heart disease, angina pectoris or other heart disease." (*Archives of Internal Medicine, 128:* 201, August, 1971).

3. ALL ABOUT CHOLESTEROL

That cholesterol is *not* a prominent constituent of an early atheromatous plaque (and this is where the vascular trouble really begins) may be found in the most respected medical textbook of all, Cecil and Loeb's *Textbook of Medicine,* 13th edition, (Philadelphia: W. B. Saunders Company, 1971). For the classical, most widely accepted, view of how atheromas (the signs of atherosclerosis in the arteries) do occur, see the article by Dr. Norman G. B. McLetchie, a pathologist from Laconia, New Hampshire— and author of the book *Coronary Atheroma: A Diary of Discovery* —in *Roche Image of Medicine & Research,* October, 1971. The idea that blood proteins such as fibrin form the primary foundation for the atherosclerotic plaque, following some injury to the blood vessel wall, is also explained in *The Journal of Clinical Investigation, 50:* 1666, September, 1971. In a somewhat related study, it has been demonstrated that an emotionally stressful situation causes an accumulation of platelets (another *protein,* not fat, blood component) within the vessels of the heart and can cause a heart attack (a report by Dr. Jacob L. Haft, chief of the Cardiac Clinic of the Bronx Veteran's Administration Hospital, New York, to the 1972 meeting of the American College of Cardiology).

For a much more detailed but not too technical description of how cholesterol is formed in the body, and how other fatty acids are absorbed and utilized, send for the free booklet, "Lipids ... in brief," put out by Ayerst Laboratories (Medical Department, 685 Third Avenue, New York, N.Y. 10017). For much more comprehensive information on the fat composition of foods, and which foods contain which fatty acids (you might be surprised to learn how much unsaturated fat is in butter and meat and how much saturated fat is in cottonseed oil), check the National Research Council Publication No. 575, available from the Food and Nutrition Board of the National Academy of Sciences, Washington, D.C. 20418 (or your local congressman or senator's office if the academy ignores your request).

Should this subject be of particular interest, especially how the body absorbs and manufactures cholesterol and how it maintains a cholesterol balance, see the books *Review of Physiological Chemistry,* edited by Harold A. Harper, Ph.D. (Los Altos, California: Lange Medical Publications, 1969), and *Physiological Chemistry of Lipids in Mammals,* by E. J. Masoro, Ph.D. (Philadelphia: W. B. Saunders, 1968). A specific reference as to how man has the ability to stabilize his blood cholesterol no matter what he eats is found in the *Annals of the New York Academy of Sciences, 149:* 838, November 21, 1968. Fish oil (probably the food containing the greatest amounts of long-chain polyunsaturates) can cause an increase in one's blood cholesterol (*Nutrition, 12:* 330, April, 1963). And then there is "Cholesterol Absorption Vs. Cholesterol Synthesis in Man" (*Nutrition Reviews, 28:* 11, January, 1970.)

What happens if the body does not have enough cholesterol has been demonstrated by the Brookhaven National Laboratory (*Medical Tribune,* September 22, 1971). And for those who want to find out about "mother's milk," see the *Proceedings of the Society for Experimental Biology and Medicine, 124:* 1020, July, 1967.

Then, to document where the excessive polyunsaturates go in the body, if one attempts to reduce the blood cholesterol, see "Polyunsaturated Fats in Nutrition," a lecture given by Dr. Ralph T. Holman of, and available from, the University of Minnesota, Austin, Minnesota. Dr. Holman comments on how the measurement of blood cholesterol is a poor index of what happens inside the individual as a whole, and that there really is a question as to whether lowering one's blood cholesterol is beneficial.

4. THE UNPUBLICIZED SIDE OF THE CHOLESTEROL
CONTROVERSY

The details of the study of Roseto, Pennsylvania are found
in the article "Unusually Low Incidence of Death From Myocardial Infarction [heart attack]," published in *The Journal of the
American Medical Association, 188:* 845, June 8, 1964, with a follow-up in *The American Journal of the Medical Sciences, 254:* 385
October, 1967. The American Medical Association has also published an official policy statement which says proof that lowering
cholesterol via diet will lower the incidence and death from heart
disease is lacking (*The Journal of the American Medical Association,
194:* 1149, December 6, 1965). And in the same medical journal,
Dr. Marvin Bierenbaum has shown that the type of fat one uses
causes no difference in either blood cholesterol or in death from
coronary disease (*202:* 1119, December 25, 1967).

At the 1970 meeting of the American Heart Association, *The
New York Times* (November 13, 1970) was the only newspaper to
report that not only did heart disease experts disagree on the
desirability of a diet low in saturated fat, but also that there is a
lack of any definite evidence that a diet low in saturated fat
would have the desired effect in lowering cardiac mortality without causing any adverse effects. At this time, the medical director
of the American Heart Association, Dr. Campbell Moses claimed
the American Heart Association's emphasis was not on increasing
polyunsaturates in the diet—yet the Association's booklets and
publicity continue to stress this type of diet, and commercial
interests still use the Heart Association's printed recommendations to promote their polyunsaturate products. Dr. H. R.
Casdorph, probably the leading advocate of the drug treatment
of a high blood cholesterol, says it really does not matter if, in a

low-fat diet, the fats are saturated or polyunsaturated (*Angiology,* *21:*654, 1970). A physician in the British medical journal, *Lancet,* *2:*882, October 21, 1967, states: "Studies of serum-lipids (particularly our old friend serum-cholesterol) in volunteers and patients fed with various types of dairy products or milk fractions did not prove—at least to me—very illuminating. If anything, they merely reinforced my feeling that the relation between levels of serum-cholesterol and myocardial infarction(*heart attack*)in man is at best indirect, and perhaps at worst even downright misleading. After 20 years of trying to apply polyunsaturated fat diets to reduce heart disease, not only has coronary heart disease not diminished, but it has actually become worse."

Among the many other physicians who concur are Dr. H. B. Brown who, in the *Journal of the American Dietetic Association,* *58:*303, April, 1971, stated that the role of diet to prevent heart disease has not been confirmed. In a most detailed, comprehensive, study of heart disease in a cross-section of a select population in Georgia, Dr. John Cassel concluded that diet could *not* be the cause of heart disease which was so varied in different social classes (*Archives of Internal Medicine, 128:*887, December, 1971). This research confirmed an earlier report that the kinds of fat one eats has no relation to heart disease—at least in the same county in Georgia (*Journal of Chronic Disease, 18:*443, 1965).

The same Veterans' Administration physician who found the marked increase in cancer in patients he put on a high polyunsaturated diet has also said he could *not* prove any relationship between that diet and heart disease. He went on to say that his findings raise a red flag on any proposals to change the American diet by substituting polyunsaturates for animal fats for the entire population (*Circulation 39:*II-1, July, 1969; *The Journal of the American Medical Association, 214:*2264, December 28, 1970). Dr. Myron Texon, of New York City, also writing in the *AMA Journal* (*216:*1482, May 31, 1971) says that diet has not even been demonstrated, let alone proved, to have any relation to heart disease. He makes the point that statistical association does *not* constitute scientific proof. Even Dr. Irvine H. Page, a leading advocate for polyunsaturates, openly admits that "There is no conclusive proof that a change in one's food pattern [to polyunsaturates] alone will prevent atherosclerosis." (*Modern Medicine,* December 27, 1971). And outside of the medical journals, an insurance physician, Dr. H. Johnson, also states there is *no* relationship between diet and heart disease (*Business Management,* January, 1971).

To cite but a few of the many, many worldwide studies that absolutely contradict the idea that a diet high in saturated fats contributes to heart disease, there is the classic critical review of 98 different reports on the relationship between diet and heart disease—which showed *no* definitive relationship (*American Journal of Public Health, 60:*1477, August, 1970). In addition to Dr. George Mann's many studies of the Masai (*Journal of Atherosclerosis Research, 4:*289, 1964) and Dr. Mann's testimony that was to have been given to Senator McGovern at his diet-heart disease hearings that were cancelled: "The Saturated Vs. Unsaturated Fat Controversy, available, without charge, from the Department of Nutritional Research, 36 S. Wabash Ave., Chicago, Ill. 60603, there have been others who have confirmed Dr. Mann's observations. Dr. K. Biss reports his findings in *The New England Journal of Medicine,* April 1, 1971, and in *Pathology and Microbiology, 35:* 198, 1970. The difference between the rural and urban Swiss is reported in *The American Journal of Clinical Nutrition, 10:*471, June, 1972. That same journal also has a study of the fact there was no difference in heart disease between Trappist and Benedictine Monks whether they ate a large amount of saturated or polyunsaturated fats (*10:*456, June, 1962), and reports on the similar study of the Micronesians (*23:*346, March, 1970). The research on the diet in northwest India was in *Medical Tribune,* January 27, 1971, and then there is another study of Alaskan Eskimos who eat a diet high in saturated fats and cholesterol but have an almost total absence of heart disease (*Fat Consumption and Coronary Disease,* New York: Philosophical Library, 1958). The comparison of the Irish blood brothers living in Ireland and in Boston was reported in *Roche Image of Medicine and Research* in December, 1963, and again in June, 1972.

If nothing else, one should read the article "Newspaper Food Pages: Credibility For Sale," to understand why much of the "other side of the story" is not publicly told (*Columbia Journalism Review,* November/December, 1971).

5. THE POTENTIAL DANGERS OF
THE DIETARY TREATMENT OF HYPERCHOLESTEREMIA

An editorial in the *American Journal of Public Health, 61:* 1747, September, 1971, discussing the dietary recommendations (polyunsaturates) that are being promoted to prevent heart disease concludes its review with the statement: "Nor is the safety of the recommendations beyond dispute." With this in mind, there is the report of the original research on the toxic reactions when an excessive amount of polyunsaturates are eaten to be found in *Medical Counterpoint,* in press, and as an editorial in the *American Heart Journal,* in press.

The details of the Detroit boy who had a rupture of the spleen from eating polyunsaturates are found in the *American Journal of Medicine, 46:*297, February, 1969. And an extensive explanation of how ceroid bodies are formed, and what they signify, can be reviewed in the chapter on "Lipid Pigments in Relation to Aging and Dietary Factors," (*Pigments in Pathology,* edited by M. Wolman, New York: Academic Press, 1969).

For a more comprehensive understanding of how polyunsaturates become dangerous after they are ingested, see "Dietary Polyunsaturated Fatty Acids as Potential Toxic Factors," by Dr. James F. Mead of the University of California, Los Angeles (*Chemtech,* American Chemical Society, page 70, February, 1972). An illustrated discussion of the same subject, with emphasis on the aging effect of the polyunsaturates, is in "Where Old Age begins," by Dr. A. L. Tappel of the University of California, Davis (*Nutrition Today,* December, 1967). Dr. Tappel elaborates on this subject in much more technical detail (with particular mention of the damage polyunsaturates do to the reproductive organs and the lungs in his chapter "Lipid Peroxidation and

Fluorescent Molecular Damage to Membranes," (*Pathological Aspects of Cell Membranes,* New York: Academic Press, 1971). Dr. Henry Eyring's research on how free-radicals damage the body, especially the chromosomes, is in the August, 1971, issue of the *Proceedings of the National Academy of Sciences.* Dr. Lissy F. Jarvik, of Columbia University College of Physicians and Surgeons in New York City, has linked mental decline to chromosome damage (*Chronic Disease Management,* June, 1972). Incidentally, there is a fascinating report on the effect of saturated and unsaturated fat on the ability to learn, especially while under stress; animals on a saturated fat diet performed better, (*Psychological Reports, 29:* 79, 1971).

An increase in polyunsaturated fats as a cause of many different diseases can be found in papers by Denham Harman, M.D., Ph.D., with special emphasis on aging (*Journal of The American Geriatrics Society, 17:*721, August, 1969 and *20:*145, April, 1972; the *Journal of Gerontology, 26:*451, 1971; *Lancet, 2:*1116, November 30, 1957; *Atherosclerosis,* Proceeding of the Second International Symposium, New York: Springer-Verlag, 1970). Liver damage from polyunsaturates has been shown by Dr. Nicholas R. Di Luzio, of Tulane University in New Orleans (*Modern Medicine,* June 14, 1971), Dr. W. O. Caster (*Life Sciences, 9:*81, 1970), and Dr. S.A. Norkin (*Archives of Pathology, 83:*31, January, 1967). Evidence of liver damage directly from the use of corn oil is in the *Archives of Pathology, 82:*596, December, 1966. Details of the toxicity of corn oil, including death, are in *The Journal of Clinical Pharmacology,* page 137, May/June, 1969.

The potential dangers of giving polyunsaturates to infants is reported in *The Journal of the American Medical Association, 214:* 1783, December 7, 1970, and in *The New England Journal of Medicine, 279:*1185, 1968.

The American Academy of Pediatrics report on *not* changing the diet of children, to eliminate milk on an experimental basis, first appeared in *Pediatrics,* February, 1972. It was reiterated in *American Family Physician* for September, 1972, with attention called to the fact that it was the Inter-Society Commission for Heart Disease Resources that made the experimental, but possibly dangerous, dietary change recommendation. What has rarely been reported is that this Commission is part of the government's Regional Medical Programs with the American Heart Association serving as the fiscal agent. In reality, the American Heart Association is using government funds to promote its own unproved ideas.

Although polyunsaturated fats, when heated, polymerize (the more technically correct term, but not one familiar to most physicians), it is not wrong to say that they also become more saturated. The Chairman of the Executive Committee of the National Safflower Council, who is also an executive of Pacific Vegetable Oil Company (Saffola Margarine), admits that resaturation is accomplished through oxidative polymerization (*The Washington Post,* March 23, 1971).

Three distinct warnings against having more than ten percent polyunsaturates in the diet come from William B. Kannel, M.D., the Director of the "Framingham Study," (*Nutrition Today,* May/June, 1971); D. S. Frederickson, M.D., one of the discoverers of lipid testing, (*British Medical Journal, 2:*187, April 24, 1971); and W. E. Conner, M.D. (*Modern Medicine,* November 30, 1970).

That an excess of polyunsaturates in the diet causes a significant increase of polyunsaturated fats in the body tissues has been reported by Dr. W. Stan Wilson (*The American Journal of Medicine, 51:*491, October, 1971) and Dr. William Insull, Jr. (*American Journal of Clinical Nutrition,* page 17, January, 1970). Dr. Wilson also showed that the uric acid levels of all his experimental patients rose significantly. For additional information on the relationship of uric acid to heart disease see *Lancet, 2:*358, February 15, 1969, and *Internal Medicine News,* November 15, 1971.

It would be impossible to list all of the scientific reports that show the damage caused by eating an excess of polyunsaturated fats, but a representative sampling seems in order. Where these fats cause impaired growth may be found in *Lipids, 1:*254, July, 1966; *Journal of the American Oil Chemists' Society, 36:*638, December, 1959; *Journal of Nutrition, 71:*45, May, 1960, *Nutrition Reviews, 15:*346, September, 1957; and in the chapter "Toxicity of Heated Fats," from *Symposium on Foods: Lipids and Their Oxidation,* Westport, Conn: Avi Publishing Co., 1962. Dr. Fred Kummerow, who wrote this piece, also discusses the increase in diarrhea and the question of increased cancer. Dr. Hans Kaunitz has written about decreased growth with enlarged livers along with death of his animals in a few weeks if he used ten percent polyunsaturates in the diet to almost immediate death when he raised the amount to 20 percent (*Journal of Nutrition, 55:*577, April, 1955 and *Journal of the American Oil Chemists' Society, 33:*630, December, 1956). The study reporting the polyunsaturated oil turning to varnish in the intestine is in the *Journal of Nutrition, 60:*13, September, 1956.

While there are as many reports of the dangers from eating unheated polyunsaturated oil, as from heated oil, it does seem that heating of the oil increases its toxicity. The work of Dr. Kritchevsky, of the famed Wistar Institute in Philadelphia, where he showed an *increase* in atherosclerosis from corn oil, is summarized in *Medical Counterpoint,* March, 1969. What happens to polyunsaturates when they are heated is elaborated on in *Bulletin 662* of the Mississippi State University Agriculture Experimental Station, May, 1963. Additional data may be found in the *Journal of the American Dietetic Association, 56:*130, February, 1970. A copy of the abstracts of all the papers presented at the 1972 meeting of the American Oil Chemists' Society on the subject "Biological Significance of Autooxidized and Polymerized Oils," will round out one's knowledge.

There are innumerable reports on the evident relationship between increased cancer and the use of excessive polyunsaturates. For an overall review see the chapter "Nutrition in Relation to Cancer," in the book *Advances in Cancer Research,* New York: Academic Press, 1953, and the article "Some Thoughts on Food and Cancer," *Nutrition Today,* January, 1972. The comparison between polyunsaturated fats and saturated fats and the former causing an increase in breast tumors is in Table 5 *CRC Critical Reviews in Food Technology, 1:*331, September, 1970. One of the authors is Dr. Daniel Melnick, Vice President of Best Foods division of CPC International, Inc., and the "referee" who reviewed the article is Dr. Fredrick J. Stare of Harvard. A more detailed explanation of how polyunsaturates actually cause cancer is found in the *American Journal of Medicine, 35:*143, August, 1963; *Medical Tribune,* September 29, 1971; and in the book *Hyaluronidase and Cancer,* New York: Pergamon Press, 1966. The relationship of polyunsaturates to breast cancer is discussed further in *The Canadian Medical Association Journal, 98:*590, March 23, 1968.

Since excessive ingestion of polyunsaturates has been so closely associated with an increased incidence of cancer, it might be of interest to note that American Indians in the southwestern part of the United States—whose diet is rich in saturated fats—

have an extremely low death rate from cancer. These Indians eat eggs every day and their regular diet always contains lard, cheese, regular meats other than veal, and especially variety or organ meats (*The Journal of the American Medical Association, 221:*550, August 7, 1972; *American Journal of Clinical Nutrition, 24:*1281, October, 1971).

For a general textbook of foods and cancer, see *Modern Nutrition and Disease,* Fourth edition. Philadelphia: Lea & Febiger, 1968.

As to how reliable a dietary questionnaire can be, see *The American Journal of Clinical Nutrition, 25:*91, January, 1972.

6. THE GOVERNMENT VS. THE CONSUMER
IN THE MATTER OF CHOLESTEROL

The way children are being taught to think their parents are deliberately killing them when a good nutritional breakfast is offered was reported in *The New York Times* (June 8, 1972). How effective such misleading, and even harmful, governmentally sponsored teaching is has been shown by the studies of Dr. Jane S. Lewis, professor of Nutrition at California State College, Los Angeles, who found that middle-class children especially are beginning to be deprived of the excellent egg source of protein and other nutrients because of their parent's unjustified fear of cholesterol.

The official attitude of the FDA, which is supposedly against the advertising or labeling of products to indicate they may be heart-saving—or even that they are high in polyunsaturates or low in cholesterol—is expressed in a letter from Charles Edwards, M.D., FDA commissioner, to Congressman L. H. Fountain, some of which was reported in an article in *The Washington Post* (March 1, 1971). On the matter of the FDA ignoring illegal advertising to physicians, contact Donald N. Kilburn, Assistant to the Director of the Division of Regulatory Operations, Office of Compliance, Bureau of Drugs, Rockville, Maryland 20852. Or, ask your U.S. Senator for a copy of the testimony on "Competitive Problems in the Drug Industry," Part 14, page 5723, 1969 (Hearings before the Subcommittee on Monopoly). A simplified, abridged, version of the subject of misleading advertising about polyunsaturates may be found in *Medical Counterpoint,* May, 1971.

Although the FDA claims it still does not endorse, or even indirectly support, any increased use of polyunsaturates, in 1971 its "news releases" admitted that it was supporting a new labeling law that would spur sales of these products (*Los Angeles Times,* June 14, 1971; *Supermarket News,* April 26, 1971). At the same time the FDA also admitted that its new labeling regulations would be illegal. Some related comments by Mrs. Virginia Knauer, the White House consumer advisor are in *Supermarket News,* July 19, 1971. At the same time Mrs. Knauer supports misleading advertising of polyunsaturates in newspapers, she also accuses newspapers of failing to live up to their "moral responsibility" by not rejecting deceptive advertisements (*The New York Times,* February 26, 1972).

For those particularly interested in how the courts interpret food and drug laws, see the legal case: *Pharmaceutical Manufacturers Association v. Richardson,* 318 F. Supp. 301 (D.C., Del., October 20, 1970) in any law library. And to measure the FDA's reaction when criticized by Congress see *Science, 175:*1347, March 24, 1972.

The FDA has continually been accused of being lax on enforcing violations (see the report by Dale B. Hattis, available from him at Stanford University, Stanford, California, and the article in *Private Practice,* February, 1971). For an all-encompassing critique of the way the FDA operates see "Legislation by Litigation," by Richard M. Stalvey, a former FDA official (*Nutrition Today,* March/April, 1972).

While there were many reports in newspapers and medical and trade journals about the "musical chairs" switching of the chief FDA lawyer and the chief lawyer for the polyunsaturate industry, the most comprehensive one was in the New York *Daily News* (September 1, 1971). The recently published book, *The Superlawyers* (New York: Weybright & Talley, 1972), documents the shift of these people that Congressman Benjamin S. Rosenthal of New York calls "a disgrace." For a picture of how the FDA has operated since the "musical chairs" game, see *Science,* July 28, 1972, for the article, "A Case Study of Regulatory Abdication," and then *Science,* August 11, 1972, for the article, "FDA General Counsel Hutt: A Man Trying to Serve Two Masters."

For the story of the attack against saccharin, see the FDA News Release Number 72-7 (dated January 28, 1972) and the *Federal Register* order for the same date. The FDA Internal Memo Number 72-21 (dated April 16, 1972) to its field personnel discusses how the FDA can use its "mislabeling" laws when it wants to and ignore these laws at other times. Referring again to the piece in the *Columbia Journalism Review* (November/December, 1971), you will understand how misleading food advertising is not only willingly accepted by newspapers, as their most profit-making device, but you will even see the open admission of how newspapers offer "free food promotion" if advertising is purchased. Thirty different major newspapers subscribe as a group to this money-making proposition. Should there be some "bad" news about a food product, it will rarely see print in a paper that carries commercial advertising for that food.

Another example of how the FDA turns its back on its own laws (and thinking back on the fuss the government made over the book *Calories Don't Count* because it was supposed to be misleading), take a look at the paperback book entitled *The Executive Diet,* (New York: Corinthian Editions, 1969) written by a pediatrician for grown-up executives. This book is given away (although it has a price on the cover of $1.95) at medical meetings, and doctors are told they can have as many copies as they wish by writing the Best Foods Division of Corn Products International, Inc. Needless to say the book primarily promotes Mazola oil (a Best Foods product) as a definitive prevention and treatment for heart disease—something the FDA says is illegal. Booklets given away by other polyunsaturate manufacturers such as Fleischmann's also tell you that you can prevent heart disease through the use of their product, and the FDA does nothing to stop this promotion which it says is against the law.

Insofar as advertising goes, Mazola claims to be the "highest in polyunsaturates," which it is not, but here the Federal Trade Commission (FTC) does nothing to uphold its prescribed duty to stop such false claims. The FTC will take action against Listerine saying the company falsely claims its product will prevent or lessen a cold (*The New York Times,* November 4, 1971), and it will take action against health food advertising by a sugar company that sells "Sugar in the Raw," because it says the company's product is not "organically" grown (*Los Angeles Times,* May 31, 1972). But it will do nothing about the unproven statements and claims advertised for polyunsaturated margarines and oils.

As somewhat of a summary of just how the government really acts in the matter of diet and heart disease, see the article

"Prevention of Atherosclerosis: Fact or Fiction?" (*Medical Counterpoint,* April, 1972). Here you will see just how your tax money is used to deceive you.

7. THE DAIRY INDUSTRY AND THE CHOLESTEROL CONTROVERSY

When thinking about the dairy industry, keep in mind that the nation's dairy farmers' income, as reported in 1972 by the Agriculture Department, was a record $6,800,000,000.00—and this in the face of Americans using fewer dairy products than ever. The net annual income (after all expenses) of the average dairy farmer in Wisconsin rose to $21,000.00 for 1970; more than twice what it was in 1964. From the total income, the dairy industry allocated $21,257,866.00 as "promotional" funds. It also allocated $400,000.00, or less than 2 percent of its "promotional" funds, for only 22 research projects on the nutritional value of milk and milk products, and only four of these 22 projects have any bearing on the relation of diet to heart disease.

The National Fisheries Institute in Chicago, or the California Fisheries Association in Los Angeles, will provide you with many different folders all wrongly telling you that fish has less cholesterol in it than milk. These folders were written by Dr. Fred Stare who also claims, in *Family Circle* magazine (February, 1971), that the "commonly used portion" of fish, or meat, is only *one ounce* (less than a one-inch cube or no more than two level tablespoonfuls). Even as a strict dieter, try sitting down to a dinner of only a one-inch piece of steak or chicken. But then Dr. Stare had to compare one ounce of fish to an eight-ounce glass of whole milk in order to make his cholesterol values come out as they did —to indict milk. This is the same Dr. Stare who admitted to Congress he works on behalf of the Cereal Institute, the Sugar Association, the Pharmaceutical Manufacturers Association, the Kellogg Company and Nabisco among others. (*The Washington Evening Star,* September 22, 1970). General Foods contributed $1 million toward the building that houses Dr. Stare's office and the cereal industry gives his department, at Harvard University, at least $40,000 a year (the knowledge of which caused at least one newspaper to drop Dr. Stare's food column (The York, Pennsylvania, *Gazette and Daily*).

The latest report on meat fats, and how they really affect one's cholesterol, was presented at the 1972 meeting of the American Institute of Nutrition by Dr. W. O. Caster of the University of Georgia, Athens, Georgia 30601. Two other medical papers support the fact that the primary fatty acids of meat fats have no effect on one's cholesterol (*Metabolism, 14*:776, July, 1965; *American Journal of Clinical Nutrition, 20*:475, May, 1967).

In the matter of how much of your tax money goes for dairy subsidy, especially butter, all the data is available from the Agriculture Department; a brief summary of the facts and figures, however, appeared in *The New York Times* (July 2, 1971). In addition to the in-depth article on the dairy lobby in *The Washington Monthly* (May, 1971), there are endless newspaper items on the dairy industry and political contributions, price manipulations and price supports (*The New York Times,* January 25, 1972 and February 2, 1972; *The Los Angeles Times,* February 18, 1972 and August 26, 1972.) The series of articles in the *Minneapolis Tribune* on the dairy lobby, by Frank Wright, appeared during June, 1971. Another view of the same subject appears in the book *The Great American Food Hoax* (New York: Dell Books, 1972).

The *American Medical News* for August 9, 1971 (published by the American Medical Association) first reported on the McGovern Senate hearings on diet and heart disease and told that the American Heart Association was the "sparkplug" of these hearings. Senator McGovern's actions in this matter were detailed in *The New York Times* (January 30, 1972) and in *The Washington Post* (May 28, 1972).

The American Medical Association's critique of how advertising, based on a person's fears, can build a multi-million dollar industry appeared in its publication *Today's Health* (April, 1972).

That the dairy industry is producing milk with an increased polyunsaturate fat content was published in the *Journal of Dairy Science* (February, 1972).

The dairy industry can condemn the misleading reports on cholesterol and saturated fats (see the National Dairy Council's publication *Focus* for almost any month, and especially page 7 of its Fall, 1970, *Bulletin*), and did quite a job in its comments to the Department of Health, Education and Welfare (dated October 31, 1971) on the matter of labeling fats. But at no time was this information brought to the attention of the public in a manner that was easy to understand and apply to one's diet. Yet, while the dairy industry was allegedly complaining about the proposed FDA regulations that would do nothing more than endorse poly-unsaturates, the head of the Dairy Industry Committee (the Washington lobby group) frankly admitted that the dairy industry would be better off with the regulations than without them.

8. DIET AND PHYSICAL FITNESS—YOU NEED BOTH

When one talks of diet and heart disease, the first thing that usually comes to mind is cholesterol—followed by the foods that are supposed to raise or lower cholesterol in the·blood. Such foods, if they consist of saturated fats are called "wrong" foods by the Fleischmann Margarine Company (in their booklet called *Dietary Control of Cholesterol*); a polyunsaturated fat such as theirs, however, is called the "right" kind, albeit it only contains about 20 percent polyunsaturates and has one of the lowest ratios of polyunsaturates to saturates of all commercial margarines (*Journal of the American Dietetic Association,* 56:29,1970).

The Fleischmann Company uses the American Heart Association publications to justify its stand; yet, the most recent official policy statement of the association on the diet-heart question may be found in the A. H. A.'s *Monograph Number 28* (available for $4.00 from the American Heart Association, 44 East 23rd Street, New York, N.Y. 10010). This report, subsidized by your tax money rather than from the funds donated by the public, was made specifically to advise the federal government of the problems and potentialities of drastically changing the American diet. The end-result was that there was *no* conclusive proof to justify any alteration in the type of fat people eat and that polyunsaturates have *not* been shown to prevent heart trouble. As recently as July 29, 1972, at a diet-heart disease symposium, Dr. Campbell Moses, medical director of the American Heart Association, was asked if it has *ever* been shown that heart attacks can be prevented by following the association's dietary recommendations, and Dr. Moses replied: "No."

Incidentally, the same Dr. Moses has stated that the biggest change he foresees in the therapy for heart disease is that: "patients are going to take the responsibility for change into their own hands; they will no longer wait passively for doctors to act." (*Medical Opinion,* July, 1972). Studies show that patients are already doing just that; they are increasing the amount of polyunsaturates they eat without consulting their physicians and they are subjecting themselves to all the potential dangers of this abnormal diet.

At the same time the American Heart Association—National Heart Institute diet-heart review panel was being conducted—the one whose results are referred to in *Monograph 28*—a member of that panel was telling a Congressional committee that: "Changing one's diet so fewer total calories of less saturated fat [sic], less cholesterol, and more polyunsaturated fats are consumed will lessen your chances, mine, and those of most of our fellow Americans of developing heart disease" (Testimony of Dr. Fred Stare, printed in the hearings before the House of Representatives Committee on Education and Labor, May 21-June 3, 1968). In direct contradiction to Dr. Stare's remarks, and as a consequence of the diet-heart study to which Dr. Stare contributed, Dr. Theodore Cooper, director of the National Heart and Lung Institute for whom the study was made, stated: "I would be unwilling to recommend modification of the total diet [in reference to cholesterol and polyunsaturated fats] on the basis of present information" (*Medical World News,* December 24, 1971). Again, the Framingham Study also found no discernible association between dietary fat consumption and serum cholesterol levels, as well as no evidence to show that any diet modification could prevent atherosclerosis (*Medical World News,* September 11, 1970; December 24, 1971). For more details on Dr. Cooper's attitude in this matter, see his article entitled "Arteriosclerosis: Policy, Polity, and Parity," (*Circulation, 45*:433, February, 1972).

When you do hear or read about research trying to justify the connection between saturated fats and heart trouble, as well as the alleged value of polyunsaturated fats as a therapeutic agent, be sure and look for the sponsor of that work—that is, who gave the money. As only one example, in an overall paper that condemns saturated fats, support came from Corn Products International—a prime seller of polyunsaturated products (*Preventive Medicine, 1*:49, 1972). This journal is published by the recently formed American Health Foundation whose admitted policy is to extensively change the American diet to increase polyunsaturates (American Health Foundation News Release, dated November 15, 1971). Of more than passing interest it must be noted that those who helped formulate this foundation's policy, and who are on its Committee on Food and Nutrition, include Drs. Daniel Melnick and Dorothy Rathmann, both executives of Corn Products International. The chairman of the board of trustees is also the president of Norton Simon, Inc., the leading producer of cottonseed oil, which is pointedly advertised as polyunsaturated. Officials of General Foods Corporation, and many advertising executives are also part of this group, which has just been given $2,000,000.00 of your tax money to build its research facility. (HEW News Release, dated July 10, 1972). Although this group says it is not important to understand the role of cholesterol in the diet, and that, admittedly, we do not know if a cholesterol-lowering diet will prevent heart disease, we should all eat more and more products such as those sold by Corn Products International.

There is a great deal of research on the role of vitamin E in the body, from the fact that the average person does not take in enough of this vitamin to what happens to the vitamin after the processing and preparation of foods. (*Lipids, 6*:291; *Journal of Nutrition, 81*:335, 1963). That the excessive use of polyunsaturates causes a severe vitamin E deficiency is no longer in doubt (*British Medical Journal, 2*:1538, May 27, 1961; *Lancet, 2*:711, September 25, 1971; *Journal of Laboratory and Clinical Medicine, 65*:739, May, 1965). The last reference is by Drs. Pearce and Dayton who first showed the marked increase in cancer in people who eat an excess of polyunsaturates; the reference in *Lancet* explains how the lack of vitamin E, caused by the polyunsaturates, could be the cause of the cancers. (*Journal Pathology and Bacteriology, 63*:599, October, 1951)

That the loss of vitamin E may be involved in premature aging—where you look much older than you are—is discussed in *Medical World News,* December 3, 1971. How vitamin E might slow down the aging process is clearly discussed by Dr. A. L. Tappel in *Geriatrics,* page 97, October, 1968, and *American Laboratory,* September, 1972.

How a deficiency of vitamin E can cause irreversible

sterility is found in *Science, 173*:1028, September 10, 1971. The same deficiency causes damage to the testicles and is reported in *Journal of Morphology, 56*:339, 1965. In addition to the reports of damage to the blood cells, cited in previous references, the damaging effect of polyunsaturates in the presence of air pollutants, and how vitamin E might offer protection, is noted in *Medical World News,* July 21, 1972.

The most recent summary of information may be found in the proceedings of the 1971 International Symposium on vitamin E, which probably can be obtained from any vitamin E manufacturer (*e.g.,* Eastman Kodak). The most comprehensive data on vitamin E is published in *The Summary,* available from the Shute Foundation for Medical Research, London, Ontario, Canada. It is hard to believe that anything known about vitamin E has not been reported in this annual publication.

The relationship of another vitamin, ascorbic acid or vitamin C, to atherosclerosis is discussed in *The American Journal of Clinical Nutrition, 13*:27, January, 1970. Here it is shown that atherosclerosis has been produced by creating an ascorbic acid deficiency—even in the presence of cholesterol in the blood, but with no deposits of fat in the blood vessel walls.

As one more example to show how little we really know about diet and blood cholesterol, it has been found that a diet high in fiber (such as unrefined whole wheat, chick-peas, etc.) can lower what seems to be an already normal cholesterol to half its original value. And this will occur even if the individual eats large amounts of butterfat (*Medical World News,* August 4, 1972).

To learn about the lack of any relationship between one's cholesterol and high blood pressure see *The Journal of the American Medical Association, 221*:378, July 24, 1972. This article also discusses the lack of any true relationship between one's cholesterol levels and being overweight, although *if* one does have an elevated cholesterol, it usually will become less as weight is lost. In the matter of the calorie values of food, as well as their nutrient value, the best reference is the book *Food Values of Portions Commonly Used* by Bowes and Church, Eleventh edition, Philadelphia: J. B. Lippincott, 1970.

In the matter of sexual activity as exercise, the research in this area was performed by Dr. Lenore R. Zohman, a cardiologist at the Bronx Montefiore Hospital and Medical Center in New York City.

That most margarines that claim to be polyunsaturated, and which really are not, may be found in several medical articles (*Canadian Medical Association Journal, 103*:268, August 1, 1970 and *The Journal of the American Dietetic Association, 39*:313, 1961; *56*:29, 1970. The author of the latter articles makes a point of saying that when a label says "Made with 100 percent corn oil," it is misleading because first, none of these products usually approach even 50 percent polyunsaturates, even if made from corn oil, and second, the very process of manufacturing produces a quantity of saturated fatty acids.

But should you still be wondering about whether eating cholesterol will make a real difference inside of you, keep in mind that most researchers have concluded that for every 100 mg. of cholesterol you eat (the average American eats about 600 mg. a day; an 8-ounce glass of whole milk (½ pint) contains about 27 mg. while a quarter pound of beef has only 80 mg—the same as fish) you alter your blood cholesterol only 3 mg. (*Medical Counterpoint,* page 13, November, 1970). Those who are most violently against eating any cholesterol in the diet concede that the change may reach 5 mg. in the blood for each 100 mg. of cholesterol left out of the diet. (*American Journal of Clinical Nutrition, 17*:281, November, 1965). Therefore, if you reduce the amount of cholesterol in your diet to what the American Heart Association directs, you *might* lower your cholesterol a negligible amount.

9. DRUGS, CHOLESTEROL, AND HEART DISEASE

Three overall reviews of most of the drugs now being used specifically to lower blood cholesterol may be found in AMA Drug Evaluations—1971 (First edition) published by the American Medical Association, Chicago, Illinois 60610; Dr. David Kritchevsky's article, "The Use of Pharmacologic Agents in Atherosclerosis Therapy" (*Annals of the New York Academy of Science,* page 1058, 1969); and the book *The Pills in Your Life* by Dr. Michael Halberstam (New York: Grosset & Dunlap, 1972). In the latter book there is a frank admission that even if one could lower the blood cholesterol, there is not the slightest guarantee of any effect on heart disease.

Although the references cited in the preceding paragraph mention the use of vitamins, another one, in particular, discusses vitamin C being effective regardless of diet (*Lancet,2*: 1280, December 11, 1971.)

The most complete description of each drug now being experimented with to lower cholesterol is found in what is called the "package insert," or the small folder required by law to be included in every bottle of medicine. Your pharmacist always has plenty of these, or you can find copies of them in a book entitled *Physician's Desk Reference* (PDR), published annually by Litton Industries, Oradell, New Jersey 07649. Your own physician might well let you see some of the advertising he receives about each product—which is easier to read, albeit cleverly couched in words that reveal much more than the initial impact. For example, a recent (1972) mailing to physicians advertising one cholesterol lowering drug product included the *1967* "package insert" with it—which did not reveal as many dangerous side-effects as does the latest one.

While most studies specifically show that drugs sometimes work to lower cholesterol, in comparison to diet (*Medical Tribune,* June 9, 1971), in general no matter what drug is used there is a failure to reduce the number of deaths from heart disease (Presented at the 1972 meeting of The American College of Physicians by Dr. Henry Schoch of the Veteran's Administration Hospital, Ann Arbor, Michigan, after a carefully controlled, double-blind, five year study). Where some researchers do think they might have achieved a beneficial effect from a drug, they admit that effect was independent of any change in blood cholesterol (*M.D. Magazine,* page 81, March 1972). When cholestyramine was used, the researchers also noted an increase in the cholesterol synthesized by the body as the drug prevented its normal absorption from the intestinal tract. (*Medical Tribune,* May 17, 1972).

A detailed report on most of the drugs discussed in this chapter, and how they act on heart disease is in *The Journal of the American Medical Association, 214*:1303, November 16, 1970. Those treated with female hormones had an increased amount of heart trouble, as well as embolism and phlebitis—and this was reported by the overall members of "the Coronary Drug Project;" one of whom still believes in the use of these drugs. Heart attacks in women long before the menopause have been reported in *Circulation, 44*:495, October, 1971. And, in women who have been castrated (had their ovaries removed so that they no longer produced female hormones) there was no increase in heart disease as would have been expected if the estrogen theory of heart attacks had any basis in fact (*American Journal of Cardiology, 28*:1, 1971).

There are several other, even newer, drugs being tried to see if there might be some beneficial effect on heart disease, but most do not seem to help the patient avoid further heart troubles (*Internal Medicine News,* March 15, 1972). In a few instances the blood cholesterol, with no change in diet, was lowered about 15 percent—which is really insignificant. Some other, different techniques to reduce heart disease include phlebotomy (blood-letting) and surgery to by-pass the bowel so that little food will be absorbed. (*Medical Counterpoint,* April, 1972).

The story of MER/29, referred to in the main body of this book, probably offers the best, overall, discussion of drug therapy. *In the Name of Profit* by Robert L. Heilbroner, *et al.* (New

York: Doubleday, 1972). Then, after reading about that drug, look back into the American Heart Association's journal, *Circulation* for 1960 and 1961 to see the advertising the association accepted for this product, which boldly says how safe the drug is, and how it works irrespective of diet. Also note that the primary plea for doctors to use the drug is the fact that the body produces at least ¾ of its cholesterol no matter what one eats. Contrast this approach of drug advertising to that of advertising to alter the type of fat you eat.

10. STRESS AND HEART DISEASE

Two general introductions to the role of stress in all diseases, with emphasis on heart disease, may be found in the *Journal of Clinical Endocrinology,6*:117, 1946; a much easier-to-read piece by the same author, Dr. Hans Selye, is in *Nutrition Today,* Spring, 1970. "What Stress Can Do To You," was in *Fortune,* January, 1972.

The chemical link within the body between stress and a heart attack was presented to the 1972 meeting of The American College of Cardiology by Dr. Jacob L. Haft, chief of the Cardiac Clinic at the Bronx Veterans' Administration Hospital in New York City (*Medical Tribune,* August 8, 1972). Dr. Reuben E. Kron, of the University of Pennsylvania Hospital, has researched similar findings (*Internal Medicine News,* July 1, 1971). Heart attacks in patients subjected to the "stress" of anesthesia and surgery are noted in *Geriatrics,* page 25, February, 1972.

Dr. Meyer Friedman has written a great deal on the relationship of one's personality and heart disease. A detailed description of the Type A individual will be found in *The Journal of the American Medical Association, 217*:929, August 16, 1971 and in *Hospital Practice,* October, 1971. Some of Dr. Friedman's personal comments on the subject are in *Modern Medicine,* page 56, May 31, 1971. More technical details are printed in the *Proceedings of the Society of Experimental Biology and Medicine, 131*: 228, 759, 1969.

Other reports on stress and heart disease are in *Psychothera-py-Psychosomatics, 18*:275, 1970; *Geriatrics, 27*:81, January, 1972; *Annals of Internal Medicine, 75*:1, July, 1971; *Industrial Medicine, 39*:31, September, 1970; and *The Journal of the American Medical Association, 218*:89, October 4, 1971. The relationship of heart disease to work attitude has been abstracted in *Modern Medicine,* page 117, May 3, 1971. Other references to this subject are found in the annotated bibliography for Chapter 2 and 3.

The American Heart Association's attitude toward stress is expressed in its booklet "Questions and Answers About Heart and Blood Vessel Disease," available from most local Heart Association offices. But then read "Death During Psychologic Stress," (*Annals of Internal Medicine, 74*:771, 1971), and "Health and Marriage Breakdown," (*British Journal of Preventive and Social Medicine, 25*:231, November, 1971). How emotions influence diabetes is reported in *The Journal of the American Medical Association, 219*: 1703, March 27, 1972.

A simple, but most comprehensive, review of how wine affects the body is in *Wine and Your Well-Being,* by Dr. Salvatore P. Lucia, professor of medicine at the University of California in San Francisco (New York: Popular Library, 1971). There probably is still no better, or safer, tranquilizer.

Medical textbooks may be obtained at any scientific or technical book dealer, or at a university book store.

Some of the medical publications, especially those that are more journalistic than technical, may be obtained by writing the publisher:

American Medical News
American Medical Association
535 N. Dearborn St.
Chicago, Ill. 60610

Columbia Journalism Review
700 Journalism Bldg.
Columbia University
New York, N.Y. 10027

Focus
National Dairy Council
111 North Canal Street
Chicago, Ill. 60606

Internal Medicine News
4907 Cordell Avenue
Washington, D.C. 20014

Medical Counterpoint
3 Far Hills Mall
Far Hills, New Jersey 07931

Modern Medicine
4015 West 65th St.
Minneapolis, Minnesota 55435

Nutrition Today
1140 Connecticut Ave., N.W.
Washington, D.C. 20036

Medical Tribune
110 East 59th St.
New York, N.Y. 10022

Medical World News
299 Park Avenue
New York, N.Y. 10017

Roche Image of Medicine and Research
International Medical Press
110 E. 59th St.
New York, N.Y. 10022

Science
American Association for the Advancement of Science
1515 Massachusetts Ave., N.W.
Washington, D.C. 20005

INDEX

Index

A

adrenal hormones, 15
adrenalin, 98
advertising: bias in, 60; and
  cholesterol, 4, 18, 26,
  55-58, 110-112; conflicts
  in, 27; of drugs, 59, 144-145;
  effects of, 32, 43; of fats,
  145; and Food and Drug
  Administration, 37; and
  Federal Trade Commis-
  sion, 37; and Framingham
  Study, 35; misleading,
  62-64; in newspapers, 133;
  and polyunsaturates, 38,
  114
aging: and polyunsaturates,
  41-46; and skin growths,
  46; symptoms of, 45
Agricultural Research Service, 5
Ahrens, Dr. Edward H., 8
alcohol, 10, 103
alcoholism, 17
Alfin-Slater, Dr. Roslyn, 52
allergy, 104
Altschule, Dr. Mark D., 23-24,
  105-106, 111-112
American Academy of
  Pediatrics, 49, 128
American Health Foundation,
  141
American Heart Association,
  48, 50, 52, 129; on
  arteriosclerosis, 77; on
  cholesterol, 1, 21, 27, 102;
  criticism of, 58; on dairy
  foods, 67; on diet, 21, 26,
  43, 47, 77, 79, 102, 124-125,
  139, 141; influence of, 43;
  and McGovern hearings,
  137; on obesity, 79; on

polyunsaturates, 60, 77;
  public statements and
  actions by, 29; on stress,
  102, 148; on uric acid, 48
American Indians, 130-131
American Medical Association:
  on advertising, 63, 72,
  137; convention of, 59;
  "Diet, Cholesterol, and
  Heart Disease," 57-58
American Medical Association
  Council on Drugs,
  *AMA Drug Evaluation
  —1971*, 58
American Medical Association
  Council on Foods and
  Nutrition, 58
AMA Drug Evaluation—1971
  (Council on Drugs),
  58
American Milk Government
  Relations Committee,
  72
amyloidosis, 48
anemia, 11, 46-49, 87
angina, 14, 116
anti-histimine drugs, 104
A.R.S. Surveys (CEIR, Inc.),
  110
arteriosclerosis, 19, 32
Artman, Dr. Neil, R., 52-53
atherogenesis, 25, 106
atheroma, 113, 122
atheromatous plaque, 20, 22,
  122
atherosclerosis, 101; and age,
  19; in athletes, 20; and
  breast feeding, 23-24; and
  cholesterol, 20, 21, 112,
  113; and corn oil, 52, 78;
  and diet, 126, 140; and
  disease, 21, and fat, 34;

ABOUT THE AUTHORS

EDWARD R. PINCKNEY, M.D., a board-certified specialist in preventive medicine, also has post-graduate degrees in public health and law. He practices as a consultant in internal medicine in Beverly Hills, California. In the past he has held two professorial appointments. At Northwestern University College of Medicine he was in charge of preventive medicine teaching, and he was Associate Clinical Professor of Medicine at Loma Linda College of Medicine in Los Angeles, where he was Director of Audio-Visual Postgraduate Education programs for physicians (a joint project with Encyclopedia Britannica). He has written five books on medicine for the public and more than 100 scientific articles and books for the medical profession. In 1960 he was given the Honor Award in Medical Journalism by the American Medical Writer's Association. Among his many editorial duties, he was one of the editors of *The Journal of the American Medical Association,* and has been the editor, or on the editorial staff, of six different medical journals. Professionally, he is a Life Fellow of The American College of Physicians, and a Fellow of the American College of Preventive Medicine (on whose Committee on Policy and Legislation he serves).

CATHEY PINCKNEY, whose primary academic training was in psychology, has written for various television shows and motion pictures. She also authored *Granny's Hillbilly Cookbook* with Irene Ryan, who played Granny on the famous TV program, "The Beverly Hillbillies." Together, Dr. and Mrs. Pinckney have written several medical books and an encyclopedia on medicine. And, for many years they were the authors of the daily newspaper column "Mirror of Your Mind."